# Genetic Diversity and Food Security

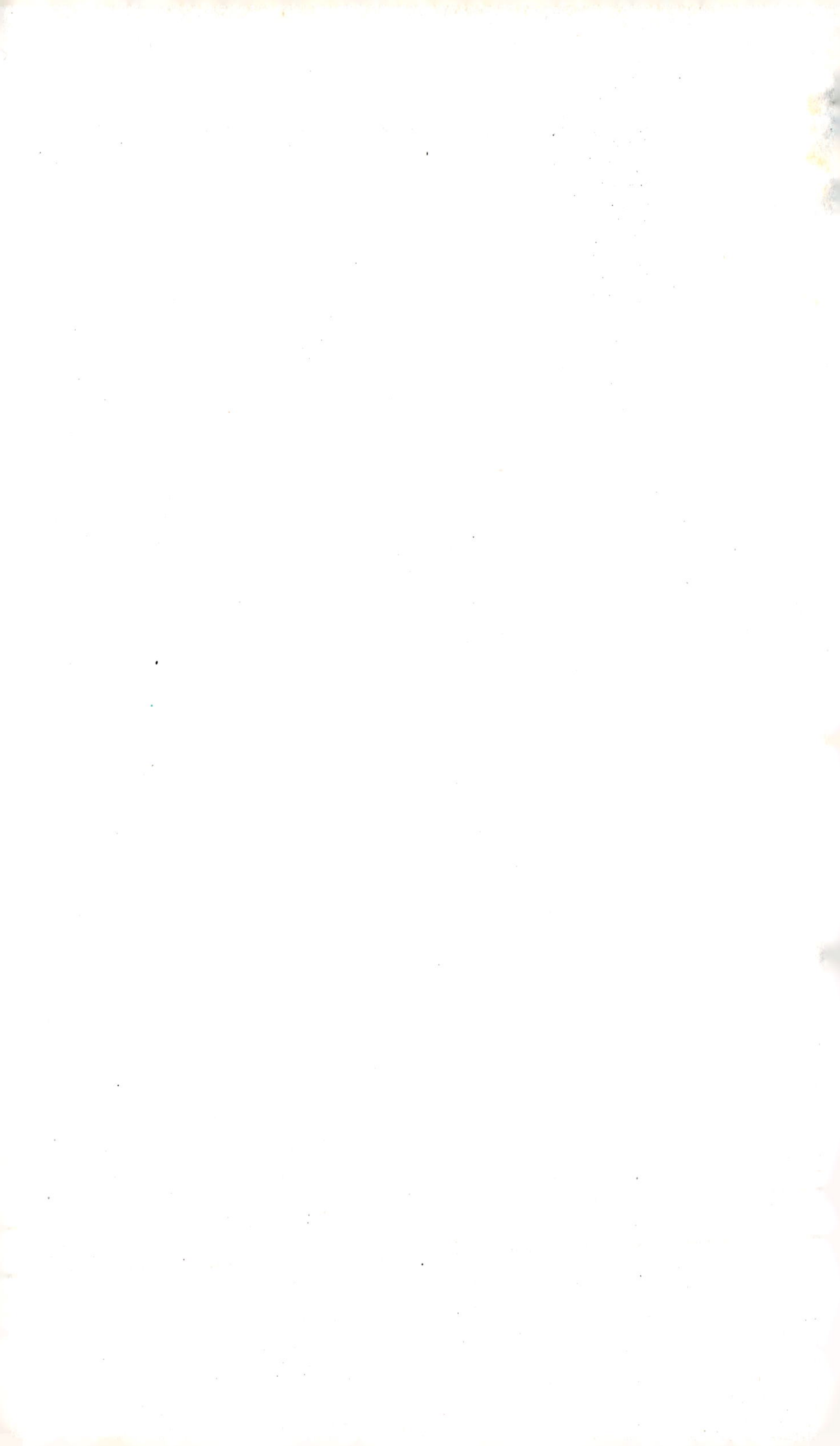

# Genetic Diversity and Food Security

*By*

**Dr. M. Lakshmi Narasaiah**
M.A., Ph.D.
*Professor of Economics,*
*Coordinator, Department of M.B.A.*
*Sri Krishnadevaraya University Post-graduate Centre,*
*Kurnool–518 002*
*Andhra Pradesh (India)*

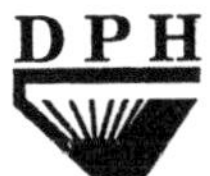


**DISCOVERY PUBLISHING HOUSE**
**NEW DELHI**

**First Published–2005**
**Reprinted-2011**
**ISBN: 81-7141-959-3**



***Published by:***
**DISCOVERY PUBLISHING HOUSE**
4831/24, Prahlad Street, Ansari Road, Darya Ganj
New Delhi–110 002 (India)
*Phone: 23279245,* • *Fax: 91-11-23253475*
**e-mail: dphtemp@indiatimes.com**

***Printed at:***
**Mehra Offset Press**
**Delhi**

# Preface

Is India's population growing disproportionately to its food supply? Will famine once again hit millions of people? Most agriculture experts agree that a Malthusian crisis is not likely to occur in the near term. The reason; the overall food situation in India has been characterized by a large increase in regional output since the famine-ravaged 1960s.

At that time, the food situation was described as "desperate" in India. Famine had plagued India's Bihar state in the sixties. International food specialists predicted further famine because food production looked as if it would lag far behind population growth. Instead, average crop yields per acre soared, thanks to the introduction of high-yielding varieties of rice and wheat and to expanded irrigation and chemical fertilizer use. It has been called the "green revolution".

**Double Role of Irrigation**

The keys to the higher food production have been irrigation, the adoption of high-yielding varieties (HYVs) of foodgrains and the increased use of modern inputs such as fertilizers. Irrigation has played a double role, it has not only helped raise yields through synergistic interaction with HYVs and fertilizers, but has also contributed to considerable increase in harvested area by enabling higher cropping intensity.

**Dr. M. Lakshmi Narasaiah**

# Contents

# 1

# Can Genetically Modified Organisms Feed the World?

The controversy over bio-technologies is raging. Advocates claim they're the only answer to malnutrition, while opponents warn that drought-resistant millet and vaccinated yams will only increase poverty. Farmers in arid and semi-arid regions of the world are anxiously waiting for rain to fall before they sow millet or sorghum, then hoe, harvest, feed their families and replenish their granaries. Meanwhile, researchers in Japanese, Chinese, Philippine, European and U.S. laboratories are making strides in sequencing the 12 chromosomes and 50,000 genes composing rice, the matrix of all grains and a staple for three billion human beings. In five to ten years, they hope to know enough to genetically modify not only rice, but millet, sorghum, manioc and sugar cane as well. The aim is to make them "naturally" resistant to drought, soil salinity, viruses, blights and other scourges.

Will these genetically modified organisms (GMOs) really guarantee "food security" in the short-term for the world's 826 million undernourished individuals? Will they help the small-scale farmers cultivating the Niger's barren, powdery soil to feed their families? In 50 years, the Earth's population will have soared to nine billion; three billion more than today. And most of the newcomers will increase the already overwhelming pressure on the southern countries' much-depleted soil. The alarm has already been sounded for sub-Saharan Africa where, unlike India and China, the population growth rate is still sky-high and the number of undernourished people is barely declining. GMO supporters say only a major revolutionary "technological leap" will enable the planet to feed all its children.

### Experimenting with Miracle Seeds

But others strongly disagree, arguing that low food production is not what causes malnutrition. There is enough to eat in the southern countries, they say. But the world's poorest people, those with neither money nor land, living in disintegrating, war-torn countries, simply have no access to food. They argue that land-use conditions must change, poor people must have access to credit and local markets and small land-owners must be freed from money-lenders. Better use could be made of traditional seeds instead of importing high-risk technology with unpredictable consequences, most of whose patents belong to giant multinationals.

Advocates of the GMO revolution work in bio-genetics laboratories, multinational seed and agrochemical companies, genome research, American foundations and some UN agencies, while most skeptics are out in the field. Adrao researchers have experience with miracle seeds. With international funding, they have developed a revolutionary variety of rice called Nerica. Genetically unmodified, it is the result of a conventional cross between a high-yield but fragile variety of Asian rice and a local variety that has had 35 centuries to adapt to Africa's stressful environment. Nerica offers tremendous possibilities. It reaches maturity in 90 days instead of the usual 120 to 150, resists insects, yield three tonnes per hectare with neither fertilizer nor irrigation - compared with 1.5 tonnes for traditional varieties - and grows like a weed. Ideally, it should improve life for hundreds of thousands of small-scale farmers who practice pluvial rice farming on plots of land ranging in size from 20 to 200 square metres and help West Africa's countries drastically cut their rice imports, perhaps even to export the grain.

### Fear and Red Tape

However, this breakthrough is having difficulty leaving the laboratory. Red tape, administrative delays and lack of communication between ministries and farmers, seed-certification organisations and rural credit institutions are to blame. A "technological leap" is not likely to help matters much.

Several African, Asian and South American countries have already passed laws regulating GMO production. But can they enforce them? Which laboratories will monitor the changes in biodiversity that might result from unforeseen crossbreeding between GMOs and related wild species? And with what funding? Who will see to it that pollen from GMOs capable of transmitting their defense mechanisms against insects and viruses do not spread? Researchers retort that it would be mistake to focus on first-generation GMOs, which are necessarily flawed. "Soon we'll see the appearance of the second, third and fourth generations, which will meet developing countries' needs better".

Bio-genetics makes it possible, for example, to insert an insect's gene into a plant or vaccines into bananas or potatoes. To create a variety of rice that needs no more water than a camel (instead of the 4,000 to 5,000 litres necessary to produce one kilo), or again, to enrich plants with vitamins and minerals and develop others that revitalize acidic soil devastated by over-farming. So why not carry out the wildest projects?

It is easy to understand the enthusiasm of certain researchers and philanthropic institutions. For example, the Rockefeller Foundation sees what it calls the biotech-driven "second Green Revolution" as a way to make up for the first one's mistakes and tragedies. True, in the 1960s, the Green Revolution helped double food production by creating high-yield varieties of wheat and rice, keeping pace with the world's population growth. But these seeds, which need plentiful inputs (irrigation, fertilizers, herbicides and pesticides), have primarily benefited farmers who could afford to invest. Africa and the poorest areas in Asia and Latin America were left out. Moreover, the results for beneficiaries, such as China and Vietnam, are mixed: traditional varieties have vanished, irrigation has increased soil salinity, and farmers have over-used herbicides and pesticides to the detriment of their health and the environment.

**Great Expectations**

Supporters of the "second Green Revolution" say GMOs should spark an explosive increase in yields without inputs and in extreme farming conditions. But will they benefit the poorest farmers? Until now, multinational agro-chemical companies converted to the "life sciences" have focused all their investments on intensive crops with close connections to industry and built a wall of prohibitively expensive patents around their discoveries. Only publicly-funded research has taken an interest in indigent farmers living in tropical areas. Strapped for cash, the public sector has been forced to sign cooperation agreements with the private sector at the risk of losing its independence.

Major biotech companies are quickly caught onto the image enhancing advantages of helping to develop GMOs for the Third World. In 2000, amid a blaze of publicity, biotech heavyweights granted the free use of 70 patents to help develop a genetically-modified variety of rice. The grain was heralded as a "miracle rice" capable of conquering Vitamin A deficiency, which kills one to two million children each year. But so far, the "golden rice" has fallen far short of expectations. The publicly-funded, Philippines-based International Rice Research Institute (IRRI) estimates that it will take five to ten years before seeds can be distributed free to farmers with annual incomes of under $ 10,000, in live with the agreements signed with industry. Furthermore, it is still unclear how much of the rice has to be consumed to make up for a Vitamin A deficiency.

For non-governmental organisations campaigning to protect the environment and preserve bio-diversity, such as the Rural Advancement Foundation International (RAFI) network, this deal "could kneecap other, low-tech and more cost-effective solutions, such as re-introducing the many vitamin-rich food plants that were once cheap and available."

**Lessons from the Past**

Will GMOs help wipe out malnutrition? The golden rice episode has set the tone for the debate. Advocates say it would be utopian to wait for a better world while existing technology can help solve the problem here and now. Some argue that lack of food is simply a problem of unequal distribution. If poor people were not poor, they could buy the food they need. This is true, but over-simplistic. There are no signs the world is about to engage in massive redistribution of wealth. First it is necessary to improve the conditions of agricultural production and soil management, keep the ground from getting hard after clearing and decrease rice imports by impoverished West African countries. All that can be achieved without GMOs, which run the risk of impoverishing bio-diversity.

# 2

# Genetic Diversity and Food Security

Maintaining a diversity of crops and varieties is a key to survival for millions of farmers living on impoverished lands. For thousands of years, farmers have used the genetic variation in wild and cultivated plants to develop their crops and raise new breeds of livestock. Genetic diversity gives species the ability to adapt to changing environments, including new pests and diseases and new climatic conditions. Plant genetic resources—that component of genetic diversity of actual or potential use to humanity—provide the raw material for breeding new varieties of crops. These, in turn, provide a basis for more productive and resilient production systems that are better able to cope with such stresses as drought or overgrazing and can reduce the potential for soil erosion. The use of genetic diversity—on-farm, through field experimentation or in sophisticated gene transfer procedures—remains arguably the best route so securing our food and that of our children.

Although science has made enormous strides in improving the world's ability to feed itself over the past three decades, we cannot afford to rest idle. Nearly 800 million people in the developing world do not have enough to eat. In these regions, the rural poor represent about 73 per cent of the people living in poverty. They often live in marginal or unsuitable farming areas, such as zones with saline soils, and conditions, or degraded or hilly areas. Often isolated from other farms and far from urban areas, many poor farmers have barely benefited from agricultural developments elsewhere. In many cases they do no have access to commercially bred high yielding crop varieties. Diversity flourishes and remains important under such conditions.

**Selections and Breeding**

Poor farmers are well aware of the relationship between the stability and sustainability of crops and crop varieties on their lands. Their management and use of a diverse range of plants has often helped them to survive under the most difficult conditions. By growing a range of different crops, farmers have a better chance of meeting their needs. These might be crops that mature at different times or that can be easily stored to ensure a stable food supply throughout the year. They may also help farmers provide a nutritionally balanced diet for their families, exploit different environment niches that exists on their land, or diversify their income sources.

Importantly, the genetic diversity contained in different varieties provides farmers with options to develop, through selection and breeding, new and more productive crops and that are resistant to pests and diseases. The result may be a vast range of local varieties of crops grown by farmers in any one area.

Not respecting diversity can incur high costs: In 18th century Ireland, where potatoes were the only significant source of food for about one third of the population, farmers came to rely almost entirely on one very fertile and productive variety, which proved susceptible to the devastating potato blight fungus. The resulting famine caused the death or emigration of more than 20 per cent of the population.

The value of diversity goes well beyond its ability to support stable production systems in marginal environments. As the world's human population rises, environmental problems (desertification, deforestation, erosion, etc.) are intensifying. Climate change, particularly global warming, could bring about drastic changes in the location of the world's agro-ecological zones. Farmers will require new crop varieties capable of producing under diverse conditions, without adding ever-increasing amounts of fertilizers and other agro-chemicals. Because of the limited scope for growth in the world's cultivated areas, each new generation of varieties will have to be more productive than its predecessors.

Much has been written about the use of genetic engineering in plant breeding. Modern molecular techniques can be used to transfer genes from one living organism to another or to change the genetic material within to produce more desirable traits. Genetic engineering has enormous potential to help solve problems that have proved intractable using conventional breeding approaches, such as developing crop varieties with in-built resistance to key pests and diseases and tolerance to stresses such as drought. However, the possible impact of these techniques, particularly on human health and the environment, is giving rise to fierce world-wide debate.

Take the case of banana and its close relative plantain, two of the developing world's most important crops. Their improvement is hindered by the sterility of most cultivars, a problem that can be addressed through genetic engineering. It is now possible to transfer gene constructs, such as those associated with disease resistance, directly into varieties with other desirable characteristics, drastically reducing the need for pesticides.

Today, research on genetic engineering is focussed on the development of commercial varieties of the world's major crops of interest to industrialized farmers. Many of the staple crops of importance to poor farmers in developing countries, such as cassava, bananas, beans and yams, have received relatively little attention. This situation is likely to continue as plant breeding is increasingly privatized and biotechnology becomes the fast-growing province of private industry. Meanwhile, the high costs of the new technologies are quickly exceeding the capacity of many, if not most, public research institutions—both in developing and developed countries—to support them. Thus, for the time being, increasing agriculture's role in the development of the world's poor is likely to continue to depend on the identification, maintenance and use of genetic diversity.

# 3

# Food First

By the time this day is over, about 40,000 human beings—mostly children—will have died from hunger, malnutrition and related causes. Today and every day the deaths will mount, reaching an annual toll of 13 to 18 million. Few of these people will have been caught up in famine or other emergencies. Most will have suffered from a "silent" assault—the kind that seldom makes the headlines, but which claims its victims just as relentlessly.

It is intolerable that such deprivation and suffering should be allowed to exist in a world of potential food plenty. Having enough food is fundamental to all else. At the most basic level, this may entail humanitarian relief to assist people in emergency situations. In the transition from relief to development, however, we must look at systems for ensuring that societies have the capacity to produce or purchase the food they need and that it is accessible to all.

Sustainable food security fuses the goals of household food security and sustainable agriculture; it requires both. It requires looking not only at the aggregate supply of food, but also at the distribution of income and land, and at other issues: Do people have enough income to buy food? Enough land to grow their own food? Does the food distribution system deliver food where it is needed? How much food is wasted due to inadequate distribution systems? What are the implications of trends in population growth for future food needs? What is the status of women in society, and what opportunities do women have to alter rapid population growth rates? What is being done to regenerate the resource base for food production? These questions need to be asked and answered in every country.

The challenge of sustainable food security is immense, and it is growing. One billion people—20 per cent of the global population—are too poor to obtain enough food to sustain normal work. Half a billion are too poor to obtain the food needed for healthy growth of children and minimal activity of adults. Today's failure to feed people, however, may be but a prologue to a much larger failure in the future. Given likely population increases, world food output must triple over the next 50 years if the world's people are to have a nutritionally adequate diet. It will be difficult enough to achieve this expansion under favourable circumstances, and conditions may be far from favourable.

For example, according to recent estimates, an area of about 1.2 billion hectares—the size of China and India combined—has experienced moderate to extreme soil deterioration since World War II as a result of human activities. Over three-fourths of that deterioration has occurred in the developing regions from causes such as overgrazing, deforestation, land cleaning, unsound agricultural practices and increased soil salinity and water logging, largely from irrigation. Other environmental threats to the agricultural resources base include loss of water and genetic resources, adverse effects of pesticides and climate change, both local and global.

At the most aggregate level, the required increase in food production could be met if production grew at the historic average, that is, at the two per cent per annum rate achieved over the past half-century. But is this realistic? To produce three times more calories, all the land currently under cultivation around the world would, within 50 years, have to attain levels of productivity as high as those exhibited by the very best cropland today.

To this challenge add the possibility of diminished returns from the technological, energy and other inputs that have made agriculture so successful. Some experts believe that most of the potential for increased output of cereals—from improved plant varieties, from increased use of pesticides and fertilizers and from expanding the area under irrigation—has already been captured.

Viewed from this perspective, the goal of achieving sustainable food security in the decades ahead emerges as one of the greatest challenges humanity has ever faced. Agricultural output must be tripled, and people must have the income to buy the food they need. The erosion of the resource base must be halted and then reversed. Failure on any of these fronts will yield unprecedented human suffering.

What will it take to achieve sustainable food security? Obviously, the effort will have to be immense, both in size and complexity. Outlined below are a few simple (but no easy) steps that are absolutely essential elements of serious effort.

First, as citizens of the world, we must all come to see sustainable food security as a fundamental aspect of global peace and human security. This goes well beyond merely denouncing the use of food as a weapon.

Second, we must adopt concrete international goals, such as reducing world hunger by half over the next 10 years. We will never achieve the goal of sustainable food security unless we aim at specific milestones and assess rigorously our progress in moving towards them.

Third, we must forge a true global partnership, a compact for sustainable food security. All countries—rich and poor—have important roles and responsibilities. There must be reciprocal responsibilities among nations, not one-way transfers.

Fourth, we must see deterioration of the agricultural resource base—terrestrial, aquatic and climatic—for what it is: a major threat to development and a major source of economic loss. Farmers are the largest group of environmental decision-makers in the world. We must ensure that they have the means to make sustainable development a reality where it counts—in the fields and fisheries.

Fifth, we must empower the people who work on the land and who keep it productive. They are in the best position to decide the most appropriate ways to graft new technology onto their own traditional knowledge of seed selection, plant protection and nutrient-cycling. Special emphasis should be given to the role of women, the main providers for two-thirds of the poorest households in the developing world, as well as the producers of 60 per cent of all food grown and consumed locally.

Sixth, we must build the capacities of developing countries, both in government and in civil society. Capacity-building means empowerment for self-reliance. It means strengthening national capacities, both inside and outside government. This is essential for recognition and analysis of problems, for decision-making on courses of action and for management of systems and processes.

Seventh, not only must we build capacity in developing countries, we must also create linkages among researchers in industrial and developing countries. This will help minimize the time lag between discovery and practical utilisation. In addition, analysts from various countries must work together to examine future food security issues with different scenarios of population growth, agricultural productivity, markets and trade, climate change, loss of soil and bio-diversity and, last but not least, political instability, in order to devise options for rational choices.

We know a good deal about how to rid the world of the scourge of hunger, and how to begin to move towards sustainable food security on a global basis. We know that economic growth and prosperity are necessary, though not sufficient, conditions for eradicating hunger. We also know that development efforts must encompass not only food production, but also socio-economic factors, including sustainable livelihoods for poor families, the implications of population growth rates, the status of women and girls and so forth. We also know that good words are not enough. Now more than ever before it is crucial that we marshal the political will to achieve our goals.

# Food Security:

## *Availability and Access to Food*

The world food situation has never been better. Enough food is being produced today that, if it were evenly distributed, no one should have to go hungry. World food production is increasing faster than population growth: per capita production increased by 5 per cent during the 1980s. Real food prices are at historic low and have been declining for some time now. Yield of major cereals have more than doubled in the past three decades. These trends have contributed to complacency in some quarters regarding the world food situation.

Yet, more than 700 million people in the developing world do not have access to sufficient food to lead healthy and productive lives. More than 180 million children are underweight. Diseases of hunger and malnutrition are widespread. The desire to satisfy food needs has, in combination with increasing population densities and inadequate agricultural intensification, led to much degradation of environmentally fragile lands, such as forests and steep hillsides.

Over the next 20-30 years, farmers and policy makers in developing countries will be challenged to provide food at affordable prices for almost 100 million more people every year—the largest annual population increase in history. Moreover, they will have to increase food production from more productive use of the land and without further degradation of natural resources: area expansion is no longer a feasible option in most of the world.

What future food security will look like depends not on exogenous factors over which we have no control but on the decisions and actions taken by the major players: households, private and public sector agencies, governments and the international community. If we continue to act as we have in the 1980s and early 1990s, more people will suffer from food insecurity. It will be because some or all of these players failed to act in an appropriate and timely manner.

### Feeding the World: Availability and Access to Food

There is enough food in the world today to feed everyone, if it were evenly distributed. Availability of daily food energy per capita in the developing countries as a whole increased by 0.7 per cent per year during the 1980s.

Twenty-five developing countries, including about half of the African countries, were unable to assure sufficient food energy (2,200 calories per person per day) for their populations at the end of the 1980s even if available food energy were evenly distributed within each country. This is down from 45 countries at the end of the 1970s.

However, available food is neither evenly distributed nor fully consumed. Availability of enough food at global, regional, or nation levels does not necessarily mean that everyone is well fed. For people to be food secure—that is, to have access at all times to the food required for a healthy and productive life—there must be both availability of food and access to food. Access to food by households (and individuals) is conditioned by poverty: the poor usually lack adequate means to secure access to food.

Over 1.1 billion people in developing countries were living in poverty in 1993, more than 500 million in conditions of extreme poverty. South Asia is the home of about 50 per cent of the developing world's poor—more than 500 million people. Another 15 per cent are found in East Asia, 19 per cent in sub-Saharan Africa, and 10 per cent in Latin America and the Caribbean. The prevalence of poverty (the proportion of each region's population that is poor) is very high—about 50 per cent in South Asia as well as in sub-Saharan Africa.

Today, there are more than 700 million people who do not have access to sufficient food to meet their needs for a healthy and productive life; they often go hungry adults and children also suffer from diseases associated with hunger and poverty. For almost one fifth of the total population of developing countries to be chronically hungry tarnishes the image of a world that is now considered food-secure because it produces enough food.

Great progress has been made in meeting food needs during the last 30 years. For instance, the number of underfed people declined from an estimated 976 million in 1974-76 to 786 million in late 1980s. But the problem is far from solved. Keeping up with increasing needs and demands due to population growth, income increases, and dietary changes is itself a formidable challenge.

Hunger and food insecurity have a significant effect on health and nutrition of both adults and children. They can lead to growth failure in children. About 184 million pre-school children in developing countries were underweight in 1994. About 55 per cent of these underweight children were found in South Asia and another 16 per cent in sub-Saharan Africa. The proportion of children that are underweight is higher in South Asia (almost 60 per cent), but it is also significant in sub-Saharan Africa (30 per cent) and Southeast Asia (31 per cent). It is worrisome that the number of underweight children in sub-Saharan Africa increased during the 1980s from 20 million to 28 million, which is particularly striking.

In addition to energy deficiencies, micro nutrient deficiencies are also widespread in the developing world. About 14 million pre-school children (under the age of five years) have eye damage as a result of vitamin A deficiency. Ten million of these children are found in Southeast Asia. Between 250,000 and 500,000 pre-school children go blind each year due to vitamin A deficiency, two-thirds of these children die within months of going blind. Many more children are mildly affected. Recently research has shown that even mild deficiencies can increase mortality significantly. Vitamin A deficiencies are closely linked to diet, which can be influenced by agricultural research and policy.

Iron deficiency affects about 1 billion people in the world, particularly children and women of reproductive age. Iron deficiency leads to anaemia, which if not checked can diminish learning capacity and increase morbidity and mortality. In the developing countries, about 370 million women between 15 and 49 years of age—42 per cent of this population group—were anaemic in the 1980s. Almost one-half were in South Asia. And there are tentative indications from South Asia and sub-Saharan Africa that the prevalence of anaemia is rising in non-pregnant adult women of reproductive ages.

In sub-Saharan Africa, this trend is undoubtedly associated with deterioration in general standards of living, including increased poverty and food insecurity. Anaemia partly arises from diets insufficient in iron, which again could be addressed through agricultural research and policy. For example, a possible reason why iron deficiency and anaemia are going up in South Asia may lie in the decrease in production of iron rich pulses during that same period, which in part reflects the larger research input into competing crops such as wheat in South Asia. This emphasises the importance of considering the effects on diet and thus on health and nutrition in setting research priorities for yield-increasing research.

South Asia is the home of about half of the developing world's hungry and food-insecure people, but this population group is growing rapidly in sub-Saharan Africa. Much of the poverty and food insecurity is in rural areas, mainly in low-potential areas such as arid zones, but urban poverty is also growing rapidly.

### Four Key Factors will Influence Future Food Production and Consumption

Global and regional food production and consumption during the next 10-20 years will be influenced by a large number of factors. Changes in the following four sets of factors are likely to be particularly important:

1. Economic growth and economic policies,
2. Population growth and urbanisation,
3. Rural infrastructure, agricultural production technology and access to modern inputs, and
4. Natural resources management and environmental considerations.

The expected impact of each of these factors on future food production and consumption is considerable.

**Economic Growth and Economic Policies**

Economic growth must resume in the developing world, especially in sub-Saharan Africa. To support such growth, it is critical to

- complete structural adjustment and economic reforms;
- remove external barriers to growth such as trade distortions and subsidies in developed countries;
- liberalize trade and remove market distortions;
- enhance access by the poor to land, capital and technology;
- expand investment in rural infrastructure, health, education and agricultural research and technology;
- facilitate sustainability in agricultural production; and
- reverse the decline in international assistance to agriculture.

Growth in real per capita income during the 1980s was disappointing for developing countries as a whole. However, the low average rate of growth covers large variations among regions. The high rates of economic growth in Asia are expected to continue through the 1990s, while incomes in sub-

Saharan Africa are expected to keep pace with population growth.

Future economic growth depends on internal policies as well as on the international policies as well as on the international environment. The extent to which current structural adjustment and economic reforms in Latin America, sub-Saharan Africa, the Commonwealth of Independent States (CIS), Eastern Europe and selected countries in Asia and the Middle East are carried to successful completion at an appropriate speed and sequence is of paramount importance for future economic growth in those countries.

Closely related to this issue is the question of the most appropriate role of the state in a market-oriented economy with inappropriate institutions, poor infrastructure and insufficient experience by the private sector in dealing effectively in a competitive market environment. Overreaction to past failures such as excessive and inappropriate state intervention may cause governments to take on a passive role where intervention is needed to assure that the markets function effectively and to deal with outside influences on the economy.

Future economic growth will also depend on the international trade environment, including trade distortions by developed countries, and access to external aid. Import restrictions for agricultural and non-agricultural products in Japan, the European Union, and the United States, along with domestic agricultural subsidies and implicit and explicit export subsidies for agricultural products, are of particular concern.

**Population Growth and Urbanisation**

If progress in economic growth is not to be undermined by rapid population growth and excessive urbanisation, effective population and migration policies are necessary to complement growth-oriented policies. Such policies must focus on.

- universal access to family planning information and technology; and

- incentives to reduce rural-urban migration, such as provision of employment in rural areas and stimulation of agricultural and non-agricultural growth in rural areas.

Although the annual growth rate is falling for the world as a whole, the population increase during the next 20-30 years, of slightly less than 100 million people a year, will be the largest ever. Approximately 97 per cent of this increase is projected to occur in the Third World, with Africa alone accounting for 34 per cent of the growth. Thus although reductions in annual population growth rates have begun to occur in Asia and Latin America, they are insufficient to counter the absolute increases. Population growth rates of these magnitudes will greatly increase the need for food and other basic necessities.

**Rural Infrastructure, Agricultural Production Technology and Access to Modern Inputs**

Continued progress in all three of these areas is critical to future food security.

- Resources must be committed to infrastructure construction and maintenance. Labour-intensive public works programmes are a viable mechanism for building roads, reforesting areas and engaging in soil conservation projects, while creating employment and income in rural areas.
- International and national agricultural research must continue to develop yield-enhancing production technology, especially in maize, millet and other crops, as well as build tolerance or resistance in crops to pests and adverse climatic conditions.
- Farmer access to modern inputs must be facilitated through provision of credit and technical assistance. Inputs must be made available to all farmers on time and in required amounts.

The importance of investments in rural infrastructure within the context of rapid urbanisation has already been established. Even without rapid urban growth, however, such investments are needed in many developing countries, particularly the poorest ones, to facilitate agricultural and rural development. Improved rural infrastructure enhances access to export markets, modern production inputs and consumer goods. It reduces marketing costs, promotes exchange between intracountry markets, reduces spatial and temporal price distortions, and, in general, increases efficiency in production and marketing.

However, while essential, effective rural infrastructure alone is not enough to assure agricultural and rural development and rapid increases in food production in developing countries. Yield-enhancing production technology is of critical importance. Although opportunities for expansion of agricultural production into lands not currently under cultivation still exist in some countries, such opportunities are so limited that they would probably not be able to counter losses of current agricultural lands to alternative uses on a global level. Furthermore, attempts to expand agricultural production into new lands would, in most cases, require large investments in technology, tools and materials and would increase the risk of land degradation and deforestation. Thus, future increases in food production must come primarily from higher yields per unit of land rather than from land expansion.

Agricultural research has successfully developed yield-enhancing technology for the majority of crops grown in temperate zones and for several crops grown in tropical zones. The dramatic impact of agricultural research and modern technology on wheat and rice yields in Asia and Latin America since the mid-1980s is well known. Less dramatic but significant yield gains have been obtained from research and technological change in other crops, particularly maize.

### Natural Resource Management and Environmental Considerations

Research, technology development, incentives and regulations are needed to prevent environmental degradation. These measures include appropriate water management policies, reduction of subsidies that encourage wasteful use of inputs, better definition of ownership and user rights to resources including land, education of farmers to encourage appropriate use of technology and resource conservation, and the provision of alternatives to resource-degrading inputs and techniques. Since poverty is a major source of degradation, poverty eradication is justified also on environmental grounds.

The recent surge in public and private concerns about negative environmental effects of economic growth and development may, if sustained, have important implications for agricultural development and future food production and consumption. Of particular concern is of the need to avoid degradation of natural resources such as land and water, as well as deforestation, water contamination and health risks associated with the use of chemicals. Since most of the current and potential resource degradation and environmental contamination result from situations in which those who cause and possibly benefit from degradation do not pay the costs, neither the market nor the individual producers and consumers are likely to incorporate preventive measures into their behaviour. Only when sufficient damage has been done to influence significantly current or future production costs will market and producer behaviour change. The state is more likely to undertake preventive measures either through publicly funded research and technology development or through incentive policies and regulations. Extensive water logging, salination and associated land degradation, and productivity losses resulting from inappropriate water management are of particular concern in large parts of Asia.

### No time for Complacency

Population growth will outstrip growth in food production in sub-Saharan Africa for a long time to come unless more is done to accelerate agricultural growth. Between now and 2000, the population will grow at more than 3 per cent a year, while food production is likely to grow at 2 per cent or less a year. By the year 2000, the production shortfall is estimated to increase to about 50 million tons of grain equivalent, up from the current level of about 14 million tons. The region will not have the necessary foreign exchange to import such large amounts of food. And African governments will not be able to count on enough food aid to make up the difference. If current trends continue, by the year 2020, Africa will have a food shortage of 250 million tons, which is more than 20 times the current food gap.

Poverty is expected to increase rapidly in the coming years. Sub-Saharan Africa's share of the world's poor is expected to increase from the current 19 per cent to about 28 per cent in 2000. Furthermore, the number of underweight children is expected to increase in the 1990's in sub-Saharan Africa.

Asian demand for cereals is estimated to grow at an annual rate of 2.1 per cent between now and the year 2000, where as food production is expected to grow at 1.9 per cent per year. Much of the production shortfall is likely to be dealt with through expanded imports and perhaps through expanded regional production in response to price increases.

In Latin America, by contrast, growth in food production is anticipated to exceed food demand growth: food production is estimated to grow by 3 per cent annually between 1990 and 2000, while food demand is estimated to grow by 2.5 per cent per year.

Large areas of land are rapidly being degraded and deforested. And the principal reasons for environmental degradation—poverty, high population growth and limited access to appropriate agricultural technology—are not being dealt with effectively.

About 700 million people are food insecure. For them the food crisis has arrived. For the 10-12 million pre-school children who died in 1994 from hunger and diseases related to malnutrition, the food crisis came and went. One-third of the pre-school children of the Third World are unable to grow to their full potential and face increased risk of death and disease.

Complacency is not in order. Clearly, Malthus underestimated the power of science to expand food production. The mass starvation that was predicted for Asia in the 1970s and 1980s did not occur because science was effectively put to work to expand crop yields. However, past yield increases came about because of people with foresight made appropriate decisions. The failure to expand investments in agricultural research and technology development during the 1980s and 1990s indicates that such foresight no longer prevails. Given the long lag time between investment in agricultural research and the resulting production increases, failure to invest today will show up in production shortfalls 10 to 20 years from now. The problems associated with environmental degradation will present themselves sooner. We must not wait until a global food crisis is upon us or until the last tree has fallen to make these investments.

## REFERENCES


1. FAO, FAO Production Yearbook.
2. FAO, "The State of Food and Agriculture 1992".
3. FAO, "Agriculture Towards 2010".
4. FAO, "The State of Food and Agriculture 1994".
5. FAO, Food Outlook (December 1994).
6. World Bank, World Development Report 1995.
7. World Bank, Global Economic Prospects and the Developing Countries.
8. World Food Programme, Food Aid in Review (Rome: WFP 1992).
9. World Bank, Global Economic Prospects and the Developing Countries, 1992. (Washington, D.C.: World Bank).

# India's Food Challenge

Is India's population growing disproportionately to its food supply? Will famine once again hit millions of people? Most agriculture experts agree that a Malthusian crisis is not likely to occur in the near term. The reason: the overall food situation in India has been characterized by a large increase in regional output since the famine-ravaged 1960s.

At that time, the food situation was described as "desperate" in India. Famine had plagued India's Bihar state in the sixties. International food specialists predicted further famine because food production looked as if it would lag far behind population growth. Instead, average crop yields per acre soared, thanks to the introduction of high-yielding varieties of rice and wheat and to expanded irrigation and chemical fertilizer use. It has been called the "green revolution".

### Double Role of Irrigation

The keys to the higher food production have been irrigation, the adoption of high-yielding varieties (HYVs) of foodgrains and the increased use of modern inputs such as fertilizers. Irrigation has played a double role. It has not only helped raise yields through synergistic interaction with HYVs and fertilizers, but has also contributed to considerable increases in harvested area by enabling higher cropping intensity.

Still, there are ominous clouds on Indian food horizon. In light of the region's high population growth, increased urban sprawl and rampant environmental degradation, there are signs that hunger problems could loom unless action is taken by Indian and international development agencies.

**Shrinking Base**

The favourable food supply situation is likely to disappear within the next decade, due to a shrinking resource base. The earlier decades had witnessed a natural resources based growth strategy as there was adequate land and water resources for development. But this is fast disappearing due to urbanisation, industrialisation and ecological degradation. We should also remember that about 50 per cent of food production is from rainfed lands and a few years of drought could alter the food security which we now enjoy. The high costs of irrigation and land development, coupled with low commodity prices, are also hampering required investments and these effects will be seen in the next decade.

By the year 2030 India will have to produce 60 per cent more rice with much fewer resources. Clearly, there will be a major challenge for scientists and policy-makers to meet the increased food demand. India's population is growing 2 per cent a year, making the challenges for regional food security a daunting task.

The solution for meeting future food demand will be breakthroughs in science and technology since yield levels have reached a plateau and are even showing signs of decline. The possibilities through biotechnology and genetic engineering are exciting and can herald another "green revolution". This is the only hope for avoiding the Malthusian dilemma.

In gauging the region's population-food squeeze, it is useful to look first at its swelling population. India, the world's second populous region, contains several states with high population growth rates.

**Ironic Problem**

Rapid population growth dilutes and impedes economic development. An increase in the population base puts greater pressure on finite resources, both financial and natural, and, in the context, worsening of income distribution, increased poverty incidence and environmental degradation.

Moreover, there is the ironic problem, that although rapid population growth increases poverty, poverty encourages larger families through its impact on access to education and decreased prospects for child survival.

If population growth is uncontrolled, the economic and social consequences are:

- ecological imbalance, with greater pressure on natural resources.
- increased urban crowding, with increases in demand for municipal services and infrastructure.
- a more unequal income distribution, particularly as labour supply outpaces job creation.
- signs of mass poverty, including high infant and child mortality rates, high levels of child malnutrition and hunger, poor school performance, unemployment and underemployment.

**Bleak Prospects**

Existing population growth rate is unsustainable, even for the relatively near future. Unless population growth rate is kept within manageable limits, the prospects for creating acceptable standards of living for low-income groups in India will be bleak.

The Indian population is growing more rapidly than ever before and will continue to do so for at least four decades. Indeed, without major technological breakthroughs and changes in patterns of consumption, even the most optimistic population growth projections are likely to be accompanied by increase in poverty, hunger and environmental degradation.

Whether we look at population, the environment or development, the next 10 years will be critical for our future. The decisions we make or don't take will widen or narrow our options for a century to come. They could decide the fate of the earth as a home for human beings.

# 6

# Food for the Billions

Will there be enough food to feed 8 billion people who will live on earth in 25 years' time? Surprisingly, few people, at least in the industrialised countries, seems to be overly concerned with this question. Whereas the world conferences on the environment, on women, human rights or social issues which were held in recent years were preceded and accompanied by intensive public debate, food does not seem to be a burning issue. Don't we have mountains of surplus food, people ask. Do we not have to pay our farmers to leave their land idle in order not to add to the glut on the world markets? And hasn't the Green Revolution ended famine even in countries like India which used to be a synonym for hungry people? So where is the problem?

The advance made in agricultural production since beginning against a background of imminent crisis are indeed remarkable. In only 20 years, yields of major crops like rice, maize and wheat in developing countries went up by 80 per cent, outpacing even the rapid increase in population. But this growth in yields has slowed down in recent years, and the aim of "food for all" is once again becoming elusive. About 800 million people still do not have access to enough food to meet their basic daily needs, nearly 200 million children suffer from protein and energy deficiencies, 88 countries—44 of them in Africa—have a deficit in food production.

Everyone wants to increase food security. The definition is that "food be available at all times, that all persons have means of access to it, that it be nutritionally adequate in terms of quantity, quality and variety, and that it be acceptable within the given culture". To achieve this goal, more food must be produced—much more, because we must not only adequately feed the 5.8 billion people already on earth, but also the additional two billion who will be added to world population in the next 25 years. Critics argue that the problem is not one of production alone, but one of poverty elimination. People are not hungry because there is no food, but because they have no money to buy it, these critics say. Available resources must be better distributed to end hunger in the world.

However, even if we succeed to eliminate poverty in the next few decades—a feat which appears highly unlikely—there would still be the need to boost production, because with rising incomes people also want to eat more and better food including meat. As can already be observed in the countries of East Asia, the newly acquired wealth leads to higher consumption levels which puts additional strains on available resources are getting scarcer. Agricultural lands are being degraded at alarming speed by erosion, salinity, desertification or disappear altogether due to urban or infrastructure development. It has been estimated that 40 per cent of productive land now has diminished capacity to supply benefits to humanity due to direct human impacts of land use. Water for agricultural purposes is getting scarcer almost everywhere, and there are hardly any land reserves to be brought into production to widen the agricultural base.

In this situation, there is no alternative to increasing and improving production from the existing land area. This can only be done through research which finds the best varieties which will bring the highest yields at the lower cost to the environment. Sustainable agriculture is the key notion—one that maintains bio-diversity, uses as little chemical inputs as possible and does not over-exploit water and soil resources.

In recent years, agricultural research has been neglected partly because of the erroneous belief that with mountains of meat and lakes of milk further production increases were not desirable. Since global grain production has stagnated and world stocks have reached an alarmingly low level last year, there has been a noticeable change of mind. To raise the awareness among governments around the world that promotion of agriculture is urgent if hunger is to be avoided in the next century.

Important work is already being done by the international agricultural research institutes which promoted the Green Revolution in the sixties and seventies and are now again in the forefront of finding solutions to the daunting task of feeding 8 billion people by the year 2020. The International Rice Research Institute (IRRI) in the Philippines, the Maize and Wheat Research Institute (CIMMYT) in Mexico or institutes like ICARDA in Syria and ICRISAT in India which work on agriculture in semi-arid and dry areas, are all seeking solutions to the problem of raising production while at the same time preserving the environment. These institutions as well as national agricultural research institutes need all the support from the public and, of course, appropriate funding, to help them accomplish their task.

The scientists are optimistic that they can develop the varieties and farming systems which will allow mankind to feed everyone on earth well into the next century. But the task is not for the scientists alone. An economic and political order must also be in place which makes it possible to eradicate poverty and allow everyone to enjoy the benefits that science can offer. Feeding the billions is, therefore, not only a scientific, but first and foremost a political.

# 7

# Less Food Security in the South

Combating hunger and poverty is the central point of Bread for the World' s mandate. In our view, that is not so much about the quantity of food produced in the world. On the one hand, it's about its fair distribution and, on the other, the access of poor people to chances of jobs. Put another way, it's to do with access to purchasing power. In the case of agriculture, that is bound up with the question of how food is produced. Whether the technologies applied maximize employment or replace work with capital.

### "Hunger Through Surplus"

The question of production, employment and distribution are tied closely to the general conditions for development. It is certainly not exclusively external economic conditions which account for hunger and under-development. Structural deficits, political conditions and wrong policies in Third World countries have become increasingly clear. However, it can still be noted that global economic framework conditions remain enormously important for the development of agriculture in the Third World.

Twenty years ago, Bread for the World publicly expounded the thesis "Hunger through surplus" and had to take much criticism for it—above all from agro-economists. But since then the contradiction between the ever-growing mountains of agricultural surpluses in the northern hemisphere and the increasing dependence on food imports of the South has become ever more apparent. Out of 120 poor developing countries, 107 today are net importers of food.

The North's surpluses of dairy products, grain, beef and sugar—which because of their production costs are exorbitantly expensive—thrust their way on to world market and destroy local supply systems (which are cheap because of subsidies), regional trade flows and the sales possibilities of potential Third World agro-exporters. Thus, the surpluses contributed to the situation that in many developing countries a policy of neglecting local agriculture can be continued with impunity.

Initially, the promise to work on the yawning gap between hunger and surplus in the world was upfront on WTO agenda. But the pattern of explanation was well simplified. It said that surpluses arose only in those countries which supported their agriculture positively and, in fact, partly excessively. And that agricultural deficiencies in countries of the South were caused mainly by deprivation of resources and capital. However, the concept of not only reducing neglect of agriculture in the South but also its oversubsidising in the North to a sensible degree and thereby eliminating their distortions of world markets had a great intellectual attraction. At any rate, it promised more justice in agriculture.

### Subsidies Can Make Sense

To avoid misunderstandings, we have nothing against the support of agriculture in Europe. Above all not when it is done for social, ecological or agriculturally beneficial reasons.

On the contrary, agriculture's important role for food security, the sustainable handling of natural resources, the settlement of rural areas and the social function of family farms justify a special position for it in economic life, including protection and support.

But that must not be carried so far that surpluses are produced with the help of dubious production methods and then dumped on the world market at markedly less than cost price, causing incalculable damage in the poor countries. On the other hand, purposeful promotion of rural development is a prerequisite and model for greater self-sufficiency worldwide, especially in Third World countries.

### Complementary Functions of World Markets

The poor countries of the South have no alternative than to become self-sufficient in food. The World markets can at best assume complementary functions. The countries would take indeterminable risks if they integrate themselves completely in the world markets, and thereby wanted to make themselves dependent upon global agro-markets. These are and will remain extremely unreliable factors that are conditioned by enormous fluctuations in prices and quantities. The powerful, and in many cases obscure, influences of multinational concerns, the manifold political interventions in the agricultural scene in most countries, and the dangers of social and ecological dumping.

But when we now look at the results of the WTO, we are disappointed. The development question and the balancing of hunger and surplus are finally no longer on the agenda. Programmes to increase food production in the poor countries were not the priority of the negotiations. The liberalisation of agro-policies in the developing countries would have meant making the disadvantaging of their farmers the subject of international negotiations. That did not happen.

On the contrary, the concepts developed with an eye on the reform of agricultural policy in the North, which target the reduction of the support level, are to be transferred to the South without questions. To be sure, there is a whole number of exemptions for the poorest developing countries. But the WTO results have also set the trend there, namely the dismantlement of subsidies. We cannot understand how such a thing can be demanded as a policy programme, especially for Africa. Support for African agriculture is largely absent, i.e. there is absolutely nothing to dismantle. That's why many international conferences repeatedly emphasize the need for these countries to achieve a greater degree of self-sufficiency in food by stronger support of their agriculture.

**Agro-Dumping**

Certainly, some changes have been made in the North's agro policy system which will also have positive impacts on world agricultural markets. However, also here we must express our disappointment. Agricultural dumping will continue. The only difference will be the new policy instrument of direct transfer of income instead of subsidised grain prices. The opening of markets in future will hardly go beyond the current preference conditions.

The entire set of W.T.O. agreements, however, bears the imprint of the two agricultural superpowers, the USA and the European Union, which make mutual concessions and coordinate their agricultural policies. But one hears nothing about the target of freeing the world agricultural market from unnecessary distortions and ensuring justice. The intention of the agro-superpowers was solely to defend their global market shares.

The development aid agencies cannot close their eyes to these problems. On the contrary, in future they must make very much greater efforts in suggesting better goals, programmes and instruments which are capable of forming a policy that can then be included in the agenda of the next round of negotiations. We may perhaps have slept a bit through the past WTO talks. Therefore it is even more important that we get very much more involved from now on.

# Food Production

During the last 25 years, world agriculture successfully expanded food production faster than population growth. This can continue for the next 25 years and beyond, if appropriate action is taken. Although world food stocks are currently low and grain prices high, the world is not about to run out of food. We can produce enough food for future generation if we choose to do so.

The widespread food insecurity, unhealthy living conditions and abject and absolute poverty in many developing countries are already threatening global stability. Failure to assure sustainable food security will foster the very conditions that will further destabilise and polarise the world in the year to come with tremendous consequences for all people.

## The Basic Facts

Poverty is widespread in developing countries, with over 1.1 billion people living on a dollar a day or less per person. Human resource development in developing countries is lagging: 1 billion people lack access to health services, 1.3 billion do not have access to adequate sanitation systems and one-third of primary school enrolls drop out by Grade 4. Natural resources, upon which future food production depends, are being degraded at alarming rates: almost 2 billion hectares of land have been degraded in the past 50 years, about 180 million hectares of forests have been converted to other uses during the 1980s, marine fisheries are collapsing around the world and regional and seasonal water shortage afflict many developing countries. Improved appropriate technology is essential to increase productivity. Yet, low-income food deficit developing countries are grossly underinvesting in agricultural research and many are reducing their support.

It calls for sustained action in six priority areas. First, we must selectively strengthen the capacity of developing country governments to perform appropriate functions such as establishing or clarifying property rights, promoting private sector competition in agricultural markets and maintaining appropriate macroeconomic environments. Predictability, transparency and continuity in policy making and enforcement must be pursued.

**Investing in People**

Second, we must invest more in poor people in order to enhance their productivity, health and nutrition. It is not only unethical but economically wasteful that a large share of the world's population is malnourished, illiterate, sick and without access to productive resources. Access to primary education, primary healthcare, reproductive care and family planning information, and clean water and sanitation must be assured for all people. Access by the poor to productive resources and remunerative employment must be improved. Empowerment of women must be supported.

Third, we must accelerate agricultural productivity. Agriculture is the lifeblood of the economy in low-income developing countries. In those countries, it provides up to three-quarters of all employment and half of all incomes. There are very strong links between agricultural productivity increases and broad-based economic growth in the rest of the economy. Agriculture is an engine of growth in low-income developing countries. National and international agricultural research systems must be mobilised to develop improved technologies focused on developing countries, and extension systems must be strengthened to disseminate the improved technologies and techniques. Low-income countries currently spend less than 0.5 per cent of the value of agricultural production on agricultural research compared to 2 per cent spent on agricultural research in middle and high-income countries. An increase of agricultural research expenditures in low-income countries to at least 1 per cent of the value of a agricultural output is urgently need with a longer term target of 2 per cent. National agricultural research must be supported by a vibrant international agricultural research system that undertakes research with large international benefits applicable across boundaries. Current investments in international agricultural research are grossly inadequate to provide the support needed by developing countries. It is of critical importance that agricultural research result in reduced unit-costs of production. Such cost reductions will make food economically accessible to low-income consumers and permit producer incomes to increase. To assure relevance of research and appropriate distribution of responsibilities, interactions between public sector agricultural research systems, farmers, private enterprises and NGOs must be strengthened.

Fourth, we must assure sustainability in agricultural production and sound management of natural resources. Farmers, local communities and governments must be encouraged to establish and enforce systems of rights to use and manage natural resources, to improve the way water is allocated and used, to reverse land degradation where it has occurred, to reduce the use of chemical pesticides and promote integrated pest management programs and to implement integrated soil fertility programs in areas with low soil fertility. Local control over natural resources must be strengthened and local capacity for organisation and management improved. Investments in less-favoured geographical areas, that is, areas with agricultural potential, irregular rainfall patterns and fragile soils must be expanded. Most poor people in developing countries reside in rural areas, and most rural poor reside in less-favoured areas. Yet, most investments, including agricultural research investments, still focus on the more-favoured areas. If we are serious about reducing poverty and protecting the natural resource base, the balance between the less-favoured and more-favoured areas must be redressed.

Fifth, we must reduce food marketing costs in low-income developing countries. The cost of bringing food from the producer to the consumer is very high in many of these countries. Efficient, effective and low-cost agricultural markets must be developed in order to bring these costs down. Inefficient state-run firms in agricultural input markets must be phased out; investment in developing and maintaining infrastructure, especially in rural areas, must be forthcoming; policies and institutions that favour large-scale, capital-intensive market agents over small-scale, labour-intensive ones must be removed; development of small-scale credit and savings institutions must be facilitated, and technical assistance to create or strengthen small-scale, labour-intensive competitive rural enterprises must be provided.

Sixth, we must expand and realign international development assistance. Many years ago, industrialised countries had agreed to allocate at least 0.7 per cent of the gross national product (GNP) to international assistance. Most countries have not reached or do not maintain this target. Not only must the industrialised countries increase international development assistance to reach the 0.7 per cent target, but they must realign it to low-income developing countries. Also, contrary to the middle and higher-income developing countries, the poorest countries are not able to gain access to capital from the rapidly expanding international commercial capital market. Developing countries in turn must seek measures to diversify sources of external funding, stem capital flight and improve the effectiveness of the aid they receive.

# Healthcare Relief in Conflict Situations:

## *What Can we Learn from the Food Relief Experience?*

Conflicts and war occur in many of the poorest nations where populations already suffer from server ill-health. War leads to an increase in disease and to a worsening of the already fragile condition of populations. Health care itself becomes a victim of conflict. Many deaths which occur during these emergencies are not discretely related to the conflict itself but are the result of lacking access to public health services. Furthermore, conflict itself but are the result of lacking access to public health services. Furthermore, conflict contributes to the deterioration of already pre-existing structural weaknesses of the healthcare system. An example is the period of internal conflict in Uganda (1970-1986) when health services declined in the aftermath of the war due to the impact of foreign assistance and the planning vacuum in which the activities took place.

### The Impact of Conflict on Healthcare

Conflict and civil strife may lead to a major disruption of health services. This is not only a result of physical destruction but also of finding shortages since national governments increase spending on military activities. Casualties increase the demand for curative services, which can divert already limited resources from preventive care.

In the case of the Sudanese civil war a large majority of health professionals was forced to abandon rural health services and left for urban areas or neighbouring countries in order to find new employment. Entire preventive health services, such as immunisation as well as water and sanitation project collapsed leaving the population exposed to infectious diseases and epidemics. In urban areas, the gap in public healthcare provision is sometimes filled with the expansion of private services. In rural areas, private sector involvement in healthcare is rather marginal, apart from some omission hospitals or pharmacies. Therefore the non-formal healthcare sector often makes a substantial contribution towards healthcare.

With the rise internal conflicts in Africa, more people suffer from emergency situations. This also increases the influence and impact of international donors. External assistance nowadays accounts for more than 25 per cent of government health expenditure in sub-Saharan Africa.

The size of donor involvement reflects the power of international agencies to control the policy domaine. Countries in conflict or post-conflict situations are under pressure to 'rescue' their health systems and accept global policies in exchange for aid assistance and relief.

However, in the period after 1991, donor organisations tended to increase their expenditures for high profile humanitarian operations rather than ordinary development activities. This shift may reflect the increasing influence of media covering some of the conflicts. Too often, organisations intervene with ad-hoc assistance without sufficient consultation at local level.

**Donors' Perceptions in Designing Relief Interventions**

Today, in many parts of sub-Saharan Africa development assistance has virtually collapsed and has been substituted by relief assistance. The problem is that relief interventions are based on a Western construction of reality, reflecting what is desirable and necessary in times of conflict. Most interventions therefore stress physical and material needs, presuming that the social aspect of food and health is not an immediate issue to address.

The question which arises here is on who's views and perceptions these needs are based? While donors interest may be guided from the perspective of ill-health, the recipient government may be concerned with the collapse of the economy. However, any intervention needs to take into account that local knowledge and practices which are shaped by state interests as well as power relationships. The common belief that healthcare systems always collapse due to conflict is sometimes mistaken, considering the fact that today's internal conflicts are often fragmented, conflicts do not necessarily result in a breakdown of the healthcare delivery system.

Donors tend of respond with a 'package' approach and developing countries' ministries of health increasingly play a symbolic role. The evidence suggests that international organisation tend to create vertical programmes which undermine national public health programmes. Foreign interventions are technically sophisticated and reorienting healthcare towards a more curative approach. Too little attention is given to strengthen the healthcare system within its own limits, providing more appropriate technology, drugs and emphasizing the training of local health staff.

Another vital issue concerns the existence of already fragile health information systems. Agencies tend to bring their own systems which leads to further fragmentation. The local perspective on what are the 'basic needs' in physical and social healthcare usually not considered. Health relief interventions do not recognise the potential of the communities and the non-formal health sector such as healers and traditional midwives in supporting and maintaining healthcare sector presents a substantial contribution towards health. It is not the question between choosing either allopathic or traditional services, it is more the decision which kind of illness will be best treated by which practitioner. There is a need in further exploring the role of this sector particularly since this is sometimes the only service available for certain populations.

**Responding to Local Needs**

More community-based public health intervention could be vital to reduce mortality and morbidity. For example in

Somalia during the 1992 war and famine high mortality rates due to measles and diarrhea could have been prevented by involving the communities in primary healthcare activities such as immunisation and nutrition improvement.

In the African context Tigray is an example where health services had been sustained and partially expanded during the civil war against the Ethiopian government. Local government structures called Baitos promoting social and economic development. Baitos encouraged communities to establish revolving funds for drugs and medical equipment. It actually functioned as early type of community financing system.

As mentioned above, the challenge in changing healthcare relief strategies is to overcome the approach of short-term interventions, particularly in changing conflict environment where conflicts are complex and interruptions are nc loner short-term. Therefore interventions need to be linked with the process of conflict resolution to avoid healthcare or food aid being used by politically dominant groups.

**Food Relief in Conflict Situations**

Food interventions have both a survival and a production function. For example, food-for-work may be part of an income programme or food aid can be monetised to generate local currency. However, food aid has to be seen beyond the objective to fulfil nutritional goals, it also defines relationships between social groups in regard to food accessibility and how food is shared. Food aid is aiming to meet people's basic food requirements and minimising risk and severity of disease by complementing services such as basic healthcare.

In more stable political conditions where free food aid is given, it presents an income transfer by releasing income, which normally is spent on food. However, in conflict situations food relief frequently becomes part of the dynamics of conflict such as in the case of Sudan where it is used to sustain the struggle between the North and the South without resolving it. Furthermore, the military attack food supplies in the fight against rebels who depend on the support from the communities.

Health is also a matter of food security. When food insecurity coincides with conflict situations, health and survival are threatened. Food security provideds some concepts on how and why vulnerable households manage to survive in periods of hardship (coping strategies).

**Coping Strategies in African Trouble Zones**

Today, most conflicts in Africa such as the ones in the Great Lake Region, Angola or Congo cause major problems of food insecurity. They are linked to the civil wars which produce substantial social disruption as a result of massive population movements. The analysis of coping strategies showed that households respond to these conflict situations by eating less, selling livestock and land, or trying to find new sources of income.

In some emergency situations, however, such coping mechanisms may fall. In the case of the war in Mozambique food aid was vital since coping strategies were limited and people had to sell all their assets which was particularly, true for internationally displaced persons and refugees.

It has been argued that food relief bypasses local structures in favour of those qualifying on a nutrition status criterion, decided by international organisation, or it may attract populations to refugee camps to receive free food rations and thereby undermines local production. In the case of Rwanda food aid was targeted at the internally displaced and left out the local population. This can be due to donor bias in needs assessment.

Food scarcity is not always the result of civil war but its creation may be rather a political objective. An example is food relief manipulated by local elites and the military like in the case of Sudan. It can be summarised that generally relief operations often bear the risk of fueling the process of instability and violence rather than helping to contain the situation.

**Lessons from Food Relief for the Health Sector**

Through the experience of food relief in recent civil wars such as Sudan, Somalia, Mozambique, etc., there has been an increasing awareness of the economic and political context in which operations takes place. Like food relief, healthcare is a political tool which can, if not properly targeted, undermine peoples access to healthcare services. While food production is linked to food security, it is more difficult to identify factors leading to self-sufficiency in healthcare.

As mentioned above, food aid is aiming to insure survival. It also has an economic aspect, protecting household assets. Healthcare relief is targeted to assure immediate physical survival based on the importance of social health. Unfortunately, curative interventions hardly consider the socio-cultural dimension of health. Therefore it would be beneficial if healthcare interventions consider local norms and traditions. Interventions should be compatible and complement local health programmes. The emphasis should be on strengthening formal and non-formal health institutions both in service provision and training.

In food relief, distribution and needs assessment identification are controversial issues for discussion. While the programme design is shaped by donor's perceptions, the actual programmes are influenced by the priorities of some powerful leaders as well as the socio-economic and political context.

Healthcare interventions need to analyse these issues in the context of economic and political systems in order to identify the most vulnerable groups, for example populations living in areas which are more affected. Operations require a stronger involvement of communities both as users and active participants carry out and maintain public health programmes.

There is a need for a new concept to be designed which applies to chronic emergencies. In the absence of a policy framework, guidelines need to be developed in order to overcome the inconsistency in planning and implementation. Donors need to change their assumptions on which they plan their health relief responses. A starting point in improving the efficiency of these operations is to provide institutional support to local authorities and organisations and involve them in the planning and implementation of programmes.

# 10

# Population Growth and Grain Production

The relationship between the growth in world population and the grain harvest has shifted over the last half-century, neatly dividing this period into two distinct eras. From 1950 to 1984, growth and the grain harvest easily exceeded that of population, raising the harvest per person from 247 kilograms to 342, a gain of 38 per cent. During the 14 years since then, growth in the harvest has fallen behind that of population, dropping output per person from its historic high in 1984 to an estimated 317 kilograms in 1998—a decline of 7 per cent, or 0.5 per cent a year.

These global trends conceal widely divergent developments among countries, contrasts that can be seen for the world's two most populous nations: India and China. In both, grain production per person was close to 200 kilograms as recently as 1978. Since then, the figure in India has edged up slightly but still falls short of 200 kilograms, while in china production has surged since the economic reforms in 1978, with per-person output now at nearly 300 kilograms. The combination of a dramatic surge in grain production and an equally dramatic reduction in population growth has given China a large margin of safety, effectively eliminating most of its hunger and malnutrition. Meanwhile, although India has also achieved impressive gains in its harvest, these have been largely cancelled by population growth, leaving its 976 million people living close to the margin.

What has happened in China and India is the story of developing countries in general. The overwhelming majority have achieved substantial, if not dramatic, gains in their grain harvests over the last half-century. Some, such as Thailand, have combined this with a much slower growth of population, which means that agricultural gains translate into rising grain production per person. In Pakistan, by contrast, grain production per person climbed steadily for a while, but it peaked in 1981 at 186 kilograms. Since then it has been declining nearly 1 per cent a years. In effect, Pakistan's farmers are losing the battle with population growth.

The slower growth in the world grain harvest since 1984 is due to the lack of new land and to slower growth in irrigation and fertilizer use. Irrigated area per person, after expanding by 4 per cent since then as growth in the irrigated area has fallen behind that of population.

The increase in world fertilizer use has slowed dramatically since 1990, as diminishing returns to the application of additional fertilizer has stabilized use in the United States, Western Europe and Japan and slowed annual growth in world fertilizer use from 6 per cent between 1950 and 1990 to scarcely 2 per cent in recent years.

Although Malthus was primarily concerned with the additional demand for grain generated by population growth, rising affluence is also playing a role. In a low income country such as India, grain consumption per person is less than 200 kilograms per year and diets are typically dominated by a single starchy staple-rice, for instance. With scarcely a pound of grain available a day per person, nearly all must be consumed directly, leaving little for conversion into animal protein. For the average American, on the other hand, the great bulk of the 800-kilogram daily grain consumption is taken in indirectly in the form of beef, pork, poultry, eggs, milk, cheese, ice cream and yogurt. At the intermediate level, in a country like Italy, people consume 400 kilograms of grain a day. Future food price stability thus depends on expanding production fast enough to keep up with both population growth and rising affluence.

One question often asked is, how many people can the Earth support? This must be answered with another question, at what level of consumption? If the world grain harvest of 1.87 billion tons were expanded to 2 billion tons in the years ahead, it would support 10 billion Indians or 2.5 billion Americans. To answer the question of how many people the Earth can support, we first have to know the level of consumption we expect to live at.

Now that the frontiers of agricultural settlement have disappeared, future growth in grain production must come almost entirely from raising land productivity. Unfortunately, this is becoming more difficult. After rising at 2.1 per cent a year from 1950 to 1990, the annual increase in rainland productivity dropped to scarcely 1 per cent from 1990 to 1997. The challenge for the world's farmers is to reverse this decline at a time when cropland area per person is shrinking, the amount of irrigation water per person is dropping, and the crop yield response to additional fertilizer use is falling.

# 11

# Population Growth and Cropland

Since mid-century, global population has grown much faster than the cropland area. The trend is likely to continue in the next century, dropping cropland per person to historically low levels. The ever smaller per capita cropland base will make food self-sufficiency impossible for many countries, and will test the capacity of international markets to meet a growing demand for imported food.

For millennia, farmers satisfied rising food demand by bringing new land under the plow. But by mid-century cropland expansion could no longer meet the food needs of an increasingly populous and prosperous world. The 10,000 year era of steady expansion was over, and a new era began that stressed raising land productivity. As this high-yielding era shows signs of faltering, concern over the shrinking supply of cropland per person looms even larger.

Since mid-century, grain area—which serves as a proxy for cropland in general—has increased by some 19 per cent, but global population has grown 132 per cent, seven times faster. Largely as a result, grain area per person has fallen by half since 1950, from 0.24 to 0.12 hectares. Assuming that grain area remains constant, grain area per person will fall to 0.07 hectares by 2050. In crowded industrial countries such as Japan, Taiwan and South Korea, grain area per capita today is smaller than the area of a tennis court.

As grain area per person falls, more and more nations risk losing the capacity to feed themselves. Having already seen per capita grain area shrink by 40-50 per cent between 1960 and 1998, Pakistan, Nigeria, Ethiopia and Iran can expect a further 60-70 per cent loss by 2050—a conservative projection that assumes no further losses of agricultural land. The result will be four countries with a combined population of more than 1 billion whose grain area per person will be only 300-600 square metres, less than a quarter of the area in 1950.

The historical record suggests that such a small area per person will send a substantial share of a country's people to world markets for their food. Consider the experience of six countries in East Asia whose per capita grain area currently ranges from 200 to 600 square metres per person. Sri Lanka relies on imports for more than a third of its grain, while Japan, Taiwan, South Korea, and Malaysia buy more than 70 per cent of their grain from abroad. North Korea is the only one of the six that does not import heavily (it gets less than 20 per cent of its grain requirements from abroad), but its population is poorly fed-indeed, on the verge of starvation.

The concern is that population growth will push many nations—not just the four fastest-growing ones—below the 600-square metre-threshold in coming decades. In Asia alone, where grain area per person stands at 800 square metres, 16 countries are poised to cross this threshold by 2050, and many of them much sooner. As this process unfolds, the number of people who will turn to foreign markets for their food will likely jump sharply. These countries will find an increasingly tight international grain market, with nations from the Middle East, North Africa and other regions already buying a third or more of their grain overseas.

In addition to per capita losses, population growth can lead to degradation of cropland, reducing its productivity or even eliminating it from production. As a country's population density increases and good farmland becomes scarce, poor farmers are forced onto ecologically vulnerable land such as hillsides and tropical forest. In the Philippines, for example, hillside agriculture accounted for only 10 per cent of all agricultural land in 1960, but 30 per cent in 1987. Because it is highly erodible, hillside land is easily damaged; worldwide, some 160 million hectares of hillside farmland—11 per cent of cropland—were characterised in 1989 as "severely eroded." Similarly, population pressure can force peasants to overfarm the poor soils of tropical forests. After being cleared and farmed for a few years, these soils typically require fallow periods of 20-25 years, but population pressures keep poor farmers on the same land for far longer than the soils can support, cutting fallow periods to just a few years in some areas of tropical Africa and Asia.

Finally, population pressures on a fixed base of land can result in rural landlessness. In Bangladesh, for example, landlessness among rural households rose from 35 per cent in 1960 to 53 per cent in the early 1990s. Interestingly, Bangladesh is regarded as a success in slowing population expansion, as its growth rate declined from 2.8 per cent in the late 1970s to 1.5 per cent in the early 1990s. But its success came too late to prevent the increase in rural landlessness, highlighting the need to work sooner, rather than later, for population stabilisation.

# Population Growth and Oceanic Fish Catch

From 1950 until 1988, the oceanic fish catch soared from 19 million to 88 million tons, expanding much faster than population. The per capita catch increased from less than 8 kilograms in 1950 to the historical peak of just over 17 kilograms in 1988, more than doubling. Since 1988, however, growth in the catch has slowed, falling behind that of population. Between 1988 and 1996, the catch per person declined to less than 16 kilograms, a drop of some 9 per cent.

This five-fold growth in the human appetite for seafood since 1950 has pushed the catch of most oceanic fisheries to their sustainable limits or beyond. Marine biologists believe that the oceans cannot sustain an annual catch of much more than 93 million tons, the current take.

As we near the end of the twentieth century, overfishing has become the rule, not the exception. Of the 15 major oceanic fisheries, 11 are in decline. The catch of Atlantic cod-long, a dietary mainstay for West Europeans, has fallen by some 70 per cent since peaking in 1968. Since 1970, bluefin tuna stocks in the West Atlantic have dropped 80 per cent.

The next half-century is likely to be marked by the disappearance of some species from markets, a decline in the quality of seafood caught, higher prices, and more conflicts among countries over access to fisheries. Over the last two decades, a growing share of the catch has consisted of inferior species, some of which were not even considered edible in times past.

The growing scarcity of the species at the top of the food chain is reflected in rising prices. Poor people who once ate fish because they could not afford meat now find that meat is often less expensive than seafood. Although most price rises are moderate, some are extreme—going far beyond anything we could have earlier imagined. The decline of the bluefin tuna population in the Atlantic, for instance, has occasionally pushed prices for a 300-kilogram tuna above $80,000 at top-of-the-line, Sushi restaurants in Japan compete for the few of these giant fish that are available.

This growing competition for limited resources has led to ongoing conflicts among countries. The United Nations recorded more than 100 such disputes in 1997. These are evident in the cod wars between Norwegian and Icelandic ships, between Canada and Spain over turbot off Canada's eastern coast, between China and the Marshall Islands in Micronesia, between Argentina and Taiwan over Falkland island fisheries, and between Indonesia and the Philippines in the Celebes. There are "tuna wars in the northeast Atlantic, crab wars in the North Pacific, squid wars in the southwest Atlantic, salmon wars in the North Pacific, and pollock wars in the Sea of Okhotsk." Although these disputes make it into the world news only rarely, they are now an almost daily occurrence. Indeed, historians may record more fishery conflicts during one year in the 1990s than during the entire nineteenth century.

One of the consequences of modern fishing technologies, whether it is the use of drift nets or bottom-scouring fish-catch of unwanted species, this oceanic equivalent of clear-cutting is damaging fisheries on an unprecedented scale.

With the oceans now pushed to their limits, future growth in the demand for seafood can be satisfied only by fish farming. As a result, aquaculture output has increased from 7 million tons in 1984 to an estimated 26 million tons in 1977. Most of this growth in catch is based on just a few species, such as carp, which constitute most of the aquacultural harvest in China, and catfish, which dominates fish farming in the United States. As the world turns to fish farming to satisfy its needs, fish begin to compete with livestock and poultry for foodstuffs such as grain, soyabean meal and fish meal.

Given that the oceanic fish catch is apparently now at or beyond its sustainable limit, it is a relatively simple matter to determine the future oceanic catch per person. With each year, this will decline by roughly the amount of population growth, dropping to 9.9 kilograms per person in 2050, a decline to little more than half the 1988 peak of 17.2 kilograms. Those of us born before 1950 have enjoyed a doubling of the seafood catch per person, while those born in recent years are likely to witness a decline of nearly one half during their lifetimes.

# 13

# The Future of Agricultural Trade

In the Uruguay Round, countries recognised that the long term solution for agriculture did not lie in administered prices, trade restrictions, supply controls and export subsidies, but rather in open, nondistorted markets. It is the time to take bold steps towards bringing agricultural trade into the 21st century by accelerating agricultural trade reform.

There are four key areas for accelerating reforms: eliminating export subsidies; increasing market access through substantial tariff cuts and expansion of tariff-rate quotas; cutting further trade-distorting domestic subsidies; and ensuring technical standards based on sound science.

The world's farmers and ranchers are facing two difficult challenges at the dawn of the 21st century. First, they are being asked to provide more products at lower cost, higher quality, greater variety and in a safer manner than ever demanded before. Second, they are being asked to produce this abundance on a shrinking natural resources base that is often subject to government regulations. Meeting these global challenges will require unleashing the production potential of world agriculture while practicing proper environmental stewardship. The ingenuity and hardwork we usually associate with farmers will be essential to meet these challenges, but they will not be sufficient unless we further reform agricultural trade to create an environment that rewards risk and investment and encourages efficiencies.

**Today's Agricultural Challenges**

Farmers are responsible for feeding a rapidly growing

world population. And despite progress over the years, too many people still are not getting enough food. Many countries including the United States, are working vigorously to promote technological innovations to meet the need for food and fiber in the coming years. However, as important as this work is, it is only part of the solution. These technologies and the hard work of the world's farmers need a trading environment that encourages investment and efficient production, and generates economic growth to finance production and consumption needs. Long-term trends in agriculture pose serious challenges for all farmers. The same technological advances that increase yields may result in lower prices. Increasing social concerns about effect of agricultural production on the environment and living conditions result in new restrictions on farm activities. As urban dwellers and industry stake competing claims for land, water and energy, many producers find their ability to farm made ever more difficult.

Two approaches to organising the agricultural economy present a stark contrast in dealing with these challenges. One model, popular in Europe and Asia, is to retain an inward-looking agricultural system focused on supply control and government regulation geared to keeping farm prices high and, since guaranteed high prices are a drain on the treasury, to controlling production. Under this approach, bureaucrats try to assess the optimal level of national production—not so little that imports are needed and not so much that excess production; must be bought at high prices and; then dumped on world markets. This "command-and-control" structure stifles farmer efficiency and ingenuity and distorts world markets, especially as subsidised surpluses are regularly exported; and it does not address the challenge to farmers to produce food for the next century. It also ignores the interest of domestic consumers (who have to pay high internal prices) and producers in other countries (who have to compete with subsidised products). Of biggest concern is that the anti-market policies of this approach hamstring the agriculture sector from pursuing the technological advances needed to meet its future challenges.

Another approach is to place agriculture on a more market-oriented basis, particularly by removing trade barriers and reducing trade-distorting policies. Greater market orientation was the principle that actions agreed to in the last set of multilateral trade negotiations. In the Uruguay Round, countries recognised that the long-term solution for agriculture did not lie in administered prices, trade restrictions, supply controls and export subsidies, but rather in open, nondistorted markets. Now is the time to take bold steps towards bringing agricultural trade into the 21st century by accelerating agricultural trade reform.

**The Gains From Trade**

The benefit from free and fair trading of agricultural products have immediate effects on people. Eliminating trade barriers and reducing unfair competition will help ensure that farmers have incentives to produce and consumers have access to the products they desire. Liberalising agricultural trade will contribute to better resource allocation by farmers, which has conservation benefits, rewards low-cost producers, encourages efficiencies and removes the drag on economic growth.

Opening trading opportunities also increases the food security of food-importing countries by giving supplier countries the confidence required to put more land into production and to create marketing relationships. Trade provides consumers with year-round access to a greater variety of less expensive products while rewarding producers, who are able to find and meet specific consumer demands, for high-value products. In a broader context, by allowing imports that are more efficiently produced elsewhere, trade encourages specialisation in efficient agricultural and nonagricultural production.

More dramatically, trade literally saves lives. Without the international flow of food products from areas with abundant production to areas where food is scarce, many people in the world would be eating less or not at all. Trade has dynamic effects, as well, that push long-term productivity growth. For example, access to customers in overseas markets creates an incentive for technological innovation, resulting in exciting developments in improved seed varieties and production techniques. International markets also expand market outlets, raising prices and giving producers increased confidence to produce more than required merely for national needs, allowing productive farmers to not only feed their neighbours but literally feed the world.

Equally important, trade in agricultural products is becoming increasingly critical to farm and ranch incomes. Increased productivity and often times flat domestic demand increases the importance of reliable international markets. Foreign markets are not just a dumping ground for surplus products; overseas consumers value choice and quality, particularly when producers in their own country cannot meet their demands or when they are charged inflated prices. Consequently, foreign and value-added agricultural producers, raising farm-gate prices and helping support the range of agriculture-related industries.

Political reality also encourages a focus on international markets: policies based on high government guaranteed prices are ultimately politically untenable because they are hugely expensive, unresponsive to the needs of customers and producers, insensitive to environmental and agronomic realities, and a shameful waste of economic assets. Rather than farming government programs, our producers are looking for customers around the world.

While agricultural trade benefits consumers and producers alike, it is an area in which progressive reform is ardently opposed by entrenched domestic interests. Producers in some countries, cosseted by high guaranteed prices and protective tariffs, oppose any move towards greater market orientation. Intervention in the agricultural economy—measured by the Organisation for Economic Cooperation and Development by summing price supports, direct payments and other supports as a per cent of total agricultural production—has actually increased in some countries from the levels at the beginning of the Uruguay Round. In the last set of multilateral trade negotiations, countries began the process of dismantling protection and delinking farm support from production decisions. Consequently, reforms have been undertaken by some countries.

### The WTO Opportunity

The major objective in the upcoming farm talks is to accelerate the reform process initiated in the Uruguay Round. That means further substantial negotiations on tariffs, subsidies and other trade-distorting measures so that the level and direction of trade are determined by market forces, not government intervention. Four key areas are outlined below.

(i) **Export Competition:** Export subsidies are the most distorting trade tool because the level and direction of trade is directly determined by government subsidies. Today, the European Union (EU) is the only substantial export subsidizer—nearly all other countries agreed not to use, or have only limited recourse to use, export subsidies in the last round of negotiations. EU farmers, responding to domestic prices frequently twice the world price, produce more products than can be consumed in Europe, but at such high prices that they can be sold abroad only with generous subsidies. These subsidies push other competitive suppliers out of the market (which is expensive and unfair) and discourage production in countries that have a comparative advantage in agricultural production (which is wasteful and is threatening both to the environment and to future farm production needs).

In the Uruguay Round negotiations, countries acknowledged the corrosive nature of subsidies and agreed to cap and reduce their use. The upcoming negotiations should eliminate them to ensure that countries do not resort to other policy tools that allow government spending to determine winners in the marketplace. Specifically, WTO members should look closely at curbing distorted state trading agricultural export monopolies that can disguise subsidies and exert distorting market power, along with other policies used to dispose of surplus commodities on a nonmarket basis.

**(ii)** **Market Access:** Measures applied at the border to stop trade currently are the principal barrier to a freer and more open trading environment for agriculture. Market access barriers deny efficient producers the chance to compete in other markets and limit the variety and quality of products available to consumers. Opening markets and maximizing trade opportunities as fundamental principles of WTO, and we still have a long way to go in agriculture to open markets to competition.

The Uruguay Round Agreement set agricultural trade on a more predictable basis by requiring that all non-tariff measures, such as quotas and import bans, be converted to simple tariffs. While this was a necessary first step to removing trade barriers, many of the tariffs are still prohibitively high. For example, while the average tariff assessed by the United States on agricultural products is less than 5 per cent (and nearly zero for industrial products), the average agriculture tariff-rate quota (TRQ). Where only specific quantities of imports receive low duties. Many other commodities also are subject to high tariffs.

As we start the next century, higher tariffs should not stop the flow of imported agricultural products. Where TRQs remain as a transitional step before we achieve more open trade, we expect more specific disciplines on the way in which they are administered. Similarly, we need to take a hard look at agricultural state trading monopoly. Importers use of these state traders may have been justifiable when more restrictions allowed on farm trade, but in the tariff-only regime it is hard to see why a government needs to insert itself between an export and an end-user.

**(iii)** **Domestic Subsidies:** Domestic subsidy programs are often the root cause of other distorting polices. Subsidy policies that increase domestic prices above world price levels can be maintained only if price-competitive imports are restricted. Additionally, overproduction generated by high domestic prices can be sold on world markets only with export subsidies that bring the price down to the world price. While reining in distortive domestic subsidy programs has value in its own right for rationalising agricultural production, the WTO negotiations will focus on their trade-distorting elements.

In the Uruguay Round negotiations, countries agreed to distinguish trade-distorting subsidies (generally those linked to the production of a specific crop or related to price supports) from non-trade distorting subsidies (such as research and development, training and environmental production). The trade-distorting subsidies were capped, and the process of reducing allowable levels of subsidies began. This distinction is a good one: the nasty sort of subsidy that distorts markets and straitjackets producers should be cut, while programs that will increase a country's ability to produce agricultural products in the next century without distorting production incentives should not be reduced.

**(iv)** **Standards:** As WTO members make progress on cutting tariffs and subsidies, the temptation increase to disguise trade barriers as health and safety measures or other innocuous-sounding "technical standards". Moreover, when regulations purportedly designed to protect health are instead vehicles for domestic protectionism, the credibility of the entire safety apparatus of a country is put up for questioning. When good science is replaced by politics, the basis for sound health policy is undermined. Therefore, increasing government accountability by putting the emphasis on sound science for health standards should discipline disguised barriers to trade and strengthen health policy.

In the Uruguay Round, countries agreed to a set of sound principles: each has the right to maintain health and safety measures, but these must be based on sound science, backed by scientific evidence and an assessment of the risk, and be no more trade-restrictive than required to meet health goals. In practice, countries have found that these principles work well—bogus measures adopted without scientific basis have been successfully challenged in the WTO without sacrificing health concerns. Creating a supportive environment for the propagation of yield-enhancing biotech products also is critical for meeting the needs of the coming century.

**Agriculture is Different**

Agriculture occupies a special place in the national economies of most countries around the world. Farmers are responsible for feeding and clothing people. Farming also holds a powerful claim on our national cultures that calls for the preservation of rural lifestyles and values. Farm production is subject to the cruel vagaries of whether and the relentless decline in prices and increases in costs. Some people point to these factors as justifying a different treatment for agriculture in the international economy, including justifying trade-distorting agricultural policies. This is wrong-headed; societies can support farms and preserve rural communities in ways that foster choice, protect natural resources and expand trade.

Farm production in the next century cannot afford to be trapped in a static system in which prices are determined by government mandate, production decisions are controlled by central planners, and farmers are forced to produce only for local consumers. This myopic system cannot be sustained in any important agriculture producing society. Moreover, this type of system will not meet the needs of the coming century, when we will face unprecedented consumer demand and natural resource constraints.

Instead, I look forward to dynamic world of agricultural trade in which producers, exporters and retailers apply the creativity of the human mind to the natural bounty of the earth. In this "new" world, we will produce a greater amount and variety of food than ever before, feed the coming billions, sustain our environment, and unlock economic resources otherwise stifled by moribund protectionism, ultimately raising living standards around the world.

# 14

# The Indian Economy and the Cattle Wealth

Though most of the Indians are virtual vegetarians, India is home to more cattle than any other country. The country's bulging barnyard results from a complex equation of economic need and religious reverence for cows. The sum is that cattle have outstripped the resources available to feed them, and their overgrazing is racking up a sizable environmental bill. The pressure of too many cattle on too little land is turning India's beloved beast of burden into one of the country's worst environmental enemies. Many cattle exist on starvation rations, too emaciated to serve their vital roles as milk producers and draft animals. The health of Indian cattle mirrors the wealth of their owners. The stall-fed dairy herds that supply milk products to city residents are usually well-nourished, as are the draft animals of wealthier farmers. By contrast, the animals of the poor maraud through urban yards for garbage or forage any open rural land, since their owners lack both cash and land to feed them.

Hinduism has long been blamed for India's millions of hungry bovines. Under Hindu tradition, cows are revered, and laws forbid their slaughter in all but two states, Kerala and West Bengal. Recently, the leader of the Hindu Nationalist Party has even called for abolishing cow butchering by non-Hindus.

Though its contribution to India's herd size cannot be dismissed, Hinduism is much less a consideration than is the economic value of bovines to rural Indians. From the perspective of the poor, a cow is a blessing. Even a scrawny bull may be able to pull a plow—a much-needed service in India, where 70 per cent of farmland is still tilled by draft animals.

Cattle manure is invaluable for fertilizer, fuel and building mud walls. For a rural woman, a cow or a goat may be the only property she ever owns. When an animal dies, its hide can be sold for leather, its skeleton for bone meal. A cow may not be the path to riches, but it is an added hope for survival.

In a country already crowded with huge population, though, space for India's million of cattle has been steadily shrinking. Unable to divert precious cropland to fodder, poor headers instead run their beasts on the fallow lands of wealthier farmers and on common land, including village forests, wasteland and roadsides. Grazable land, however, is disappearing. Land reforms have divided common areas among farmers, irrigation has turned dry rangeland to cropland, and tractors have plowed under fallow fields. Even forestry projects have usurped former grazing land for trees. All told, India's dry regions have lost more than one-third of their common land.

On the common lands that remain, traditional village management is crumbling under population and economic pressures, so grazing is uncontrolled. As cattle overgraze grasses, they clear the way for an invasion of weeds and woody shrubs, and topsoil becomes exposed to the erosive power of wind and rain. Parched subsoil and deep gullies are all that remain in many areas.

As the condition of common lands has deteriorated, the number of goats has surged. With less discriminating palates than cattle, goats eat the weeds and shrubs on degraded areas cattle ignore. India's forests, caught between fodder and fuelwood needs, have not escaped destruction. Though state forests are usually off-limits to villagers, poor women—who collect most fodder—are driven to graze their animals on woodland grasses and illicitly cut branches for fodder. Constantly pruned back, trees eventually die, and as the canopy opens and grasses vanish, soils dry up and erode. India's deforestation and erosion problem is largely a cattle feed problem.

Relief for India's hungry cattle and battered land is not likely soon, although the loss of common land has actually compelled some peasants to give up their animals. What appears the obvious solution—killing off "excess" cattle—is constrained by legal codes and, more importantly, by poverty. Eliminating the scraggliest cattle, which belong to the poor, would make the people with the least suffer the most.

Poverty also has hampered the Government's strategy to boost each cow's productivity so that fewer are needed. For example, as part of a dairy development program dubbed Operation Flood, the Indian Government distributes European cow breeds and buffaloes that produce more milk. But villagers who can't afford low-cost fodder can hardly buy the expensive feed grains that the new animals require. On low-quality rations, the new breeds fare worse than their less-pedigreed cousins.

India's cattle will likely crowd fields and streets for years to come. There are no simple solutions, but without concerted efforts to meet the feed demands of these animals, the environmental destruction they cause may make India's favored beast more reviled than revered.

# 15

# Solving Conflicts Over Water Uses

There are few issues that have greater impact on the life of mankind and the planet as a whole than the management of our most important natural resource water. This has only been realised in detail more recently by the general public as well as by many planners and decision-makers. Around the world they have begun to appreciate the critical importance of a reliable water supply for their future survival and sustainable development. Rivers are lifelines in countries like India serving different uses such as transport, agriculture, fisheries, personal hygiene and others. Conflicts over use of water resources must be settled through better water management policies.

In many localities of the Earth water-related problems have become extremely acute, even critical. In some places they are the source of social instability and are a threat to international security. There is not the slightest doubt that, with further population increase and under the "water business-as-usual" scenario, these problems will become ever major acute, thus creating ever more instability. After decades of water waste, water pollution and inability to provide basic water services to the poor, we must fundamentally change the way we think about and manage water. We have to realise that water can no longer be considered to be a cheap and plentiful resource, which can be used, abused or squandered without much concern for further human welfare.

As fresh water is becoming scarce, that is when there is not enough water to satisfy all demands, competition develops.

Besides the well known tensions at international level over limited water supplies, there is an increasing and in many cases a far more important competition over water arising within countries, between sectors. Such competition, for instance, occurs between farmers for irrigation water and between farmers and non-agricultural users of water such as cities (including industries and power plants) and environmental concerns (recreation, fish and other wildlife). Because of this increasing competition irrigated agriculture around the world, but especially in developing countries, faces important challenges in the coming decades. On the one hand, it has to provide a major share of the required increases in food and fiber production to meet the objectives of poverty alleviation and development. On the other hand, it is threatened by water shortages arising out of increasing competition from domestic, industrial and other sectors. This situation is further worsened by dwindling financial resources available for capital expenditure as the cost of new irrigation schemes increase.

**Land under Irrigation**

On a regional basis, it is estimated that, for example, around 60 per cent of the value of crop production in Asia is grown on irrigated land. The irrigated sector performs an essential task in meeting the basic food needs of billions of people. It has provided more than half of the two most important basic staples and close to a third of all food crops. In the future, the irrigated sector will have to provide an even larger proportion of the total food output. The question arises whether irrigated agriculture will be in a position to provide the extra food needed to feed a growing population despite an increasing water scarcity and inter-sectoral competition. There is no general, no easy answer to this question. But the following implications are foreseeable.

The irrigation sector has to recognise that economic structures are dynamic and not static. The economics of many countries have undergone considerable change in the last decades. In connection with this change agriculture is losing its leading role in economic development and this is, besides other things, affecting the allocation of water resources between agriculture and other users. The same applies to many other countries around the world, especially developing countries in arid and semi-arid climates.

### New Water Policies are Needed

Because of the growing competition for ever-scarcer water resources, governments and water authorities are forced to change water policies. Objectives of the new policies are demand-decreasing and demand-shifting. Irrigated agriculture, by far the dominant water user, will be strongly affected by such policy changes.

Water has an economic value in all its competing uses and should be recognised as an economic good. Agriculture will in future not any more get water free of charge as it did in the past. Farmers will have to pay for the water, and costs will be increasing steadily over the years to come.

There will be a reduction of the role of governments in rural water projects and an increasing importance of local user groups. Experience shows that an important solution to water related problems is to give users the responsibility for developing and managing the water resource. This requires that farmers become properly organised in water user associations, able to discharge their new responsibilities and that they have security of tenure to the land they farm and irrigate.

During the recent decade growth in crop productivity in irrigated areas has slowed, and competition for water for non-agricultural uses has increased. These developments place strong demands to develop water resource policies to maintain growth in irrigated agricultural production:

- facilitate efficient allocation of water across sectors and final demands; and
- reverse the ongoing degradation of the water resource base, including the watershed irrigated land base, and water quality.

What water policies can lead to efficient increases in irrigated production while reducing resource degradation in the irrigated areas in developing countries and releasing water for growing non-agricultural demands? What policies can be implemented to conserve water in non-agricultural uses to reduce competition between sectors?

**Questions to be Answered**

Among others the following questions still have to be answered.

1. What are the implications of growing competition between agricultural and non-agricultural uses of water for the availability and productivity of water in agriculture?
2. How to use regulations, water prices, pollution taxes and effluent charges to encourage water conservation and pollution control in industries and households?
3. What are the production, equity, employment generation and income impacts of alternative water allocation mechanisms in different agroeconomic and scarcity environments? What investment and administrative costs are associated with different mechanisms? What is the impact of resource allocation methods on water use, cropping patterns, crop yields, fertilizer and other input use, capital investments, farm income, and environmental degradation?
4. What is the connection between alternative allocative mechanisms and the environmental externalities caused by irrigation, including water logging, salinisation, ground water recharge and ground water mining?
5. How will food security in low income countries be effected by changing water policies?

In the context of the growing competition for water it is important to enable policy makers to evolve a policy-mix which will result in efficient, equitable and environmentally sustainable allocation of water resources to user sectors. To achieve this, extensive research work is needed.

# Irrigation Management:

## *Facing the Challenge*

Irrigated agriculture is up against an enormous challenge. India's population continues to grow at a tremendous rate. Over the next 10 years, there will be more extra mouths to feed. Water is becoming increasingly scarce for agriculture, with conflicting demands being made on limited supplies by the domestic and industrial sectors. The most attractive irrigation sites have already been exploited. Yet, irrigated agriculture will have to deliver average output increases of at least 3.5 per cent per year if future food demands are to be met in India.

Forty years ago in the 1950s and 1960s, India has worried about its capacity to produce sufficient food to feed its growing population. Episodes of food scarcity were not uncommon. It was dreaded that millions would die of hunger. Then dawned the miracle of the "green revolution". Cereal production increased by leaps and bounds, boosted by expanded irrigation, increased fertilizer application and modern crop varieties. The vigorous response in mobilising financing towards boosting agricultural production paid off.

Given the importance of irrigation to the India's food supply and the vast resources already expanded on irrigation development, it is tragic that the actual performance of irrigation systems is so disappointingly low. In the post-green revolution era, it has become increasingly evident that the performance of irrigation systems, especially large-scale systems, is suboptimal whether measured in terms of achieving planned area targets or in terms of production potentials created by the physical works.

In many irrigation systems, the actual area irrigated is much less than the command area. Sharp inequities in water supplies between farmers in the head reaches of irrigation systems and those located downstream is another manifestation of poor performance. Investigations in the Tungabhadra Irrigation Scheme reveal that the tail-end of a major distributary commanding 25% of the total area, received approximately 20-40% of the targeted discharge while the upper reaches got more than their share.

Lack of maintenance has caused many systems to fall into disrepair, further inhibiting performance. Over time, distribution canals have become silted up, increasing the likelihood of breaching, damage to outlets and leading to salt build-up in the soil.

### Successful Farmer-managed Irrigation Systems

Farmers have long demonstrated their potential capability to manage irrigation systems efficiently. Farmer-managed irrigation systems (FMIS), also known as traditional, indigenous, communal or peoples' systems, are often classified "minor" or "small-scale" irrigation systems, although they may be found in command areas of 15,000-20,000 hectares.

Many successful farmer-managed irrigation systems which have been functioning effectively for hundreds of years represent a valuable, accumulated investment. They are also reservoirs of largely untapped irrigation management experience.

Research has revealed that FMIS contribute to the production of a significant portion of the subsistence food supply. Ground-water irrigation systems, often found in areas affected by drought, play a strategic role in promoting food security. In India ground-water development which is increasing in importance is predominantly farmer-managed. In this country an estimated 20 million hectares are already under ground-water irrigation. When mismanaged though, ground-water irrigation could impact negatively on the environment.

In addition to the hectarage under farmer-managed ground-water irrigation, farmer-managed tank irrigation systems cover about 8.5 million hectares in this country. Farmer-managed irrigation systems have also allowed intensification of agriculture to partially meet the food needs of rapidly growing populations.

### Little Awareness

Yet, despite the widespread interest in irrigation management turnover throughout India, there is very little documentation about the processes used and the results obtained from irrigation management turnover. Many policy-makers do not know how to turn over management of their irrigation institutions in an effective way. They typically have very little, if any, awareness of the range of organisational options which may be suitable under different conditions. There is an urgent need, therefore, for a systematic, comparative assessment of the range of approaches being used, constraints to implementation and the impacts on performance of transferring management to non-governmental or farmers' organisations.

Successful irrigation in the future will be that which supports much higher levels of agricultural productivity, enhances responsiveness to more diversified and dynamic crop markets, stimulates more profitable irrigated agriculture for wide number of rural poor, substantially improves water use efficiency and supports the sustainable use of scarce land, biomass and water resources.

In the coming years the irrigation sector will be in ferment, with decision makers, agency managers and farmers needing better information and strategic processes to make intelligent choices in the management of irrigated agriculture.

# Population and the Environment:

## *The Global Challenge*

As the century begins, natural resources are under increasing pressure, threatening public health and development. Water shortages, soil exhaustion, loss of forests, air and water pollution, and degradation of coastlines afflict many areas. As the world's population grows, improving living standards without destroying the environment is a global challenge.

Most developed economies currently consume resources much faster than they can regenerate. Most developing countries with rapid population growth face the urgent need to improve living standards. As we humans exploit nature to meet present needs, are we destroying resources needed for the future?

### Environment Getting Worse

In the past decade in every environmental sector, conditions have either failed to improve, or they are worsening:

**Public Health:** Unclean water, along with poor sanitation, kills over 12 million people each year, most in developing countries. Air pollution kills nearly 3 million more. Heavy metals and other contaminants also cause widespread health problems.

**Food Supply:** Will there be enough food to go around? In 64 of 105 developing countries studied by UN Food and

Agricultural Organisation, the population has been growing faster than food supplies. Population pressures have degraded some 2 billion hectares of arable land—an area the size of Canada and the US.

**Fresh Water:** The supply of freshwater is finite, but demand is soaring as population grows and use per capita rises. By 2025, when world population is projected to be 8 billion, 48 countries, containing 3 billion people will face shortages.

**Coastlines and Oceans:** Half of all coastal ecosystems are pressured by high population densities and urban development. A tide of pollution is rising in the world's seas. Ocean fisheries are being overexploited, and fish catches are down.

**Forests:** Nearly half of the world's original forest cover has been lost, and each year another 16 million hectares are cut, bulldozed, or burned. Forests provide over US$400 billion to the world economy annually and are vital to maintaining healthy ecosystems. Yet, current demand for forest products may exceed the limit of sustainable consumption by 25%

**Biodiversity:** The earth's biological diversity is crucial to the continued vitality of agriculture and medicine—and perhaps even to life on earth itself. Yet human activities are pushing many thousands of plant and animal species into extinction. Two of every three species is estimated to be in decline.

**Global Climate Change.** The earth's surface is warming due to greenhouse gas emissions, largely from burning fossil fuels. If the global temperature rises as projected, sea levels would rise by several metres, causing widespread flooding. Global warming also could cause droughts and disrupt agriculture.

### Towards a Livable Future

How people preserve or abuse the environment could largely determine whether living standards improve or deteriorate. Growing human numbers, urban expansion and resource exploitation do not bode well for the future. Without practicing sustainable development, humanity faces a deteriorating environment and may even invite ecological disaster.

**Taking Action:** Many steps towards sustainability can be taken today. These include using energy more efficiently; managing cities better; phasing out subsidies that encourage waste; managing water resources and protecting freshwater sources; harvesting forest products rather than destroying forests; preserving arable land and increasing food production through a second Green Revolution; managing coastal zones and ocean fisheries; protecting biodiversity hotspots; and adopting an international convention on climate change.

**Stabilizing Population:** While population growth has slowed, the absolute number of people continues to increase 0 by about 1 billion every 13 years. Slowing population growth would help improve living standards and would buy time to protect natural resources. In the long run, to sustain higher living standards world population size must stabilize.

18

# Population Growth and Waste

A growing population increases society's disposal headaches—the garbage, sewage, and industrial waste that must be gotten rid of. Even where population is largely stable—the case in many industrial countries—the flow of waste products into landfills and waterways generally continues to increase in coming decades, as they will in many developing countries, mountains of waste will likely pose difficult disposal challenges for municipal and national authorities.

Data for waste generation in the developing world are scarce, but citizens in many of these countries are estimated to produce roughly half a kilo of municipal waste each day. If this figure is applied to today's population, a total of 824 million tons of municipal waste is being churned out annually in developing countries. Population growth alone would boost this number to 1.5 billion tons by 2050. But waste rates tend to climb with rising incomes; a developing world generating as much waste per capita as industrial countries do today would be producing some 3.6 billion tons of municipal waste in 2050. Moreover, prosperity boosts the volume of waste as the share of plastics, metal paper and other nonorganics rises.

Local and global environmental effects of waste disposal will likely worsen as 3.4 billion people are added to global population over the next half-century. Acids from organic wastes, for example, and poisons from hazardous wastes often leach from landfills, polluting local groundwater supplies. And rotting organic matter generates methane, a greenhouse gas.

If the waste is incinerated rather than thrown into landfills, cities will have to worry about increases in cancer-causing dioxin emissions, one of the byproducts of burning garbage.

Meanwhile, today's largely unmet sanitation needs could also be greatly exacerbated by population growth. Half the world's people do not have access to a decent toilet, according to UNESCO and the World Health Organisation. Lack of sanitation is a leading cause of disease: WHO reports that half the developing world suffers from one of the six diseases associated with poor water supply and sanitation. One of these, diarrhea, is the biggest killer of children today, taking an estimated 2.2 million young lives each year. Unless the expected growth in population of the developing world is matched by an increased commitment to provide adequate sanitation, these health problems are likely to expand.

While the greatest shortage of sanitation is found in rural areas, the need is most urgent in cities, because of the greater potential there for pathogen-tainted water to sicken people on a massive scale. This urban need poses a particular challenge, because the ranks of city dwellers will swell in the next century. In contrast to global population, which is projected to increase by 54 per cent over the next half-century, cities will see much greater growth—about 128 per cent. Developing-country cities which failed to meet the sanitation needs of moré than a half-billion residents in 1994, will be hard-pressed to service more than 3 billion people who will be added to cities in the next 50 years.

Prospects for providing access to sanitation are dismal in the near to medium term. Just to keep from losing ground, the rate of provision of service to urban dwellers needs to more than double in Asia. In Africa, it would have to increase by 33 times. And to achieve full coverage by 2020, service provision would have to triple in Asia and increase by 46 times in Africa. Despite the attention focused on sanitation, governments have not demonstrated the will to meet this growing challenge.

# Saving the Planet:

## *Imperialism in Green Garb?*

Developing countries feel that protecting the world's resources is just another way for rich nations to retain the upper hand in the international trade game. For nearly a decade, international efforts to address global environmental concerns have been frustrated by a deep rift in perceptions between rich and poor countries. Economists and environmentalists in developing nations argue that the North almost exclusively drives the agenda for environmental negotiations. Under the pretext of saving the planet, they say, the industrialised world is wielding a new brand of dominance, "ecoimperialism."

Developing countries like India and China continue to resist global environmental protocols, like the 1989 Montreal Accord to cut the production of CFC gases (used, for example, in refrigerators) by 50 per cent, or the Clean Development Mechanism (CDM), part of the climate change negotiations initiated under the 1997 Kyoto Protocol.

The spectre of imperialism is likely to vitiate the next round of climate change talks in Bonn (Germany) when policymakers finalise the terms on which the CDM will be implemented. Negotiated by industrialised countries to gain some flexibility in meeting the emission reduction targets pledged in Kyoto, few issues in recent environmental diplomacy are proving as contentious.

Critics say the mechanism is the latest in a string of attempts to dominate poor countries, which are being virtually "bribed" so that rich nations can continue business as usual. By financing forestry schemes and other energy-efficient projects, industrialised countries could exploit the mechanism to avoid reducing their own greenhouse gases. Environmentalists fear this could turn the Amazon and other primeval forests into "carbon sinks" to absorb pollution, but with side effects which disregard the development needs of southern countries.

**Lopsided Negotiations**

The Northern bias continues to dominate discussion of the global climatic crisis. The threat to the atmospheric canons has been building over centuries mainly because of industrial activity in the North. Yet, discussions seems to focus more on developing countries; the North refuses to assume extra responsibility for cleaning up the atmosphere. No wonder the Third World cries foul when it is asked to share the costs.

The 1989 Basel Convention, for instance, imposed restrictions on trade in scrap metals and recyclable materials, claiming they were hazardous to the environment. Economists say it prohibits poor countries from competing in the lucrative world market for computer parts, scrap metal and recyclable products.

Other examples of trade restrictions are cited. In the early 1990s, Malaysia and Indonesia fought to overturn an ecolabelling law introduced by Austria ostensibly to safeguard the Asian rain forests. Austria refused to import timber that was not from sustainable managed forests, but no such curbs existed for wood from temperate areas. The protectionist flavour of the measure was overt, and Austria eventually revoked it.

In other trade-environment disputes over the last decade, the United States has been accused of protectionism in banning the import of Mexican tuna because dolphins were getting ensnared and killed in nets meant for the fish. Shrimp from India, Pakistan, Thailand and Malaysia, which paid no heed to seaturtle protection, were similarly banned in 1996.

The sanctions may have been motivated by a desire to protect dolphins and turtles, but the poorer countries claimed that they were a pretext for suppressing competition in the global fish market.

**A Green Agenda to Stop Growth?**

Rules restricting trade through the Basel Convention or attempts to ban genetically modified foods are designed to exclude poorer countries from world markets. Other voices in the South, however, argue that environmental controls like the CDM are not at all bad. Developing countries, say experts, will receive $5 to $17 billion to fund climate-friendly technologies. The CDM gives us an opportunity to invest in projects that promote sustainable development. If incidentally they also reduce emissions, we shouldn't quarrel with the fact.

# The Trade Related Intellectual Property Rights (TRIPS) Agreement and the Developing Countries

The basic norms of free competition established in the nineteenth century induced legislators to provide relatively weak forms of intellectual property protection. Often innovators could rely only on such factors as lead time, reputation for quality and continuing technical improvements to maintain their foothold in the market.

Undermining this outlook were two developments that led to the inclusion of intellectual property issues in the World Trade Organisation (WTO). First, the rise of knowledge-based industries radically altered the nature of competition and disrupted the equilibrium that had resulted from more traditional comparative advantages. Second, the growing capacity of manufacturers in developing countries to penetrate distant markets for traditional industrial products forced the developed countries to rely more heavily on their comparative advantages in the production of intellectual goods than in the past. Market access for developing countries thus became a bargaining chip to be exchanged for greater protection of intellectual goods within a restructured global market place.

Since 1986 the developed countries' drive for extraterritorial protection of intellectual property rights has largely ignored the competitive capabilities of developing countries with respect to intellectual goods, and it has also downplayed these countries' rights to preferential treatment under existing rules. At the same time, the logic of multilateral trade negotiations skews the pre-existing North-South conflict over intellectual property rights by introducing the prospects of trade concessions in unrelated fields. Intellectual property rights constitute but one of many variables that bear on competitive capacity and the transfer of technology in general.

### Primary Intellectual Property Regimes

#### *Patents*

The extension of patentability to virtually all types of technology recognised by developed patent systems, the prolongation of patent protection to a uniform term of twenty years, and legal recognition of the patentee's exclusive rights to import the relevant products could adversely affect developing countries whose existing patent laws fall below these standards. In practice, however, the competitive status of any given developing country in a post-TRIPS world will depend in part on the level of foreign direct investment it attracts and on the benefits that strengthened intellectual property rights bring to domestic innovators.

Competition under stronger patent regimes requires developing countries to adopt legal means of narrowing the scope of foreign patent monopolies and of encouraging local entrepreneurs either to work around the claimed inventions or to develop improvements suited to local conditions. To this end, local entrepreneurs should exploit technical information in disclosures published abroad; patent authorities should exercise all of the claims limitations practiced abroad; and domestic courts should strictly interpret the doctrine of equivalents. Legislative enactments of utility model laws would provide additional incentives to adapt foreign inventions to local conditions and to improve them further.

Moreover, unpatented traditional technologies will often remain suitable for local needs, and the resulting products may be sold at lower prices than imported products of patented technologies. Entrepreneurs in developing countries should also be prepared to exploit unpatented applications of applied scientific know-how in such advanced technologies as biogenetic engineering and computer programme-related innovation

In time, increased direct investment by foreign patentees could enable developing-country licensees who exploit their natural advantages, especially low labour costs, to succeed on both domestic and export markets where non-licensees were unable or unwilling to venture in the past. Familiarisation with the benefits of the patent system should stimulate greater investment in domestic research and development and in technological innovation.

The gradual extension of patents to new technologies such as computer programmes and bio-genetic engineering without the emergence of agreed international minimum standards creates both opportunities and risks for the developing countries. While the developed countries enjoy unique advantages in biotechnology that only become available to developing countries as a consequence of stronger patent systems, some developing countries may find their own competitive status enhanced by the provision of proprietary rights, including plant breeders' rights, though others may not. The patenting of bio-genetic advances decreases the scope for reverse-engineering and could also increase the costs of doing business in key sectors of some developing economies, notably agriculture. As regards information technologies, reliance on copyright and trade secrets at the international level appears less unfavourable to the developing countries' prospects than patents, for reasons that are set out below. However, the tendency to patent software could diminish these prospects by posing limits to reverse engineering and to the attainment of the interoperability, and this trend adds to the overall costs of disseminating information goods.

To the extent that patented technology is not made available on reasonable terms or that un-wholesome economic dependencies actually arise, developing countries will have to consider measures to restore the competitive balance that are consistent with the TRIPS Agreement. For example, the agreement allows compulsory licenses when the rights holders fail to licenses patented technology "on reasonable commercial terms". It also provides other bases for defensive regulatory action by emphasizing "the transfer and dissemination of technology to the mutual advantage of producers and users" and the need "to promote the public interest in sectors of vital importance to socio-economic and technological development".

Measures to restrain abuse of intellectual property rights as authorised by the Paris Convention also remain available under the TRIPS Agreement, which expressly empowers developing countries to deal with licensing practices that "adversely affect the international transfer of technology".

Finally, the agreement specifically preserves the right of all states to "adopt measures necessary to protect public health and nutrition and to promote the public interest in sectors of vital importance to socio-economic and technological development, provided that such measures are consistent with the provisions of this agreement".

### Trademarks and Geographical Indications

The TRIPS provisions give pre-existing norms greater specificity while softening the use requirement and eliminating both compulsory licenses and local linkage requirements. These provisions also subject the international regime of trademarks and unfair competition to more stringent enforcement measures, including border controls against imports of counterfeit goods.

As a result, developing countries will need to reassess the pro-competitive functions of trademarks in open economies while addressing questions of abuse in a more direct fashion. They should insist on receiving the technical cooperation and aid that the TRIPS Agreement envisages for the purpose of defraying administrative and enforcement burdens.

Governments should consider policies and incentives that encourage enterprises to establish their own market identities through appropriate trademarks and foreign firms to allow licensees to adapt more of the licensed products for both domestic and export needs under local trademarks.

**Copyrights**

Authors in many developing countries are very active in both domestic and foreign markets. It nonetheless remains true that the balance of trade in cultural goods favours exports from developed countries. This imbalance could increase under the TRIPS Agreement, which generally applies the international minimum standards of the Berne Convention, plus selected standards from the Rome Convention on neighbouring rights.

While efforts to implement these standards is mandatory, developing-country authorities should familiarise themselves with the extent to which the scope of copyright protection varies from country to country, in the absence of authoritative legal limitations recognised by international law. Carefully framed public-interest exceptions may further reduce the overall costs of a TRIPS Agreement without violating international copyright norms. Moreover, the revised Berne Convention already provides for compulsory licenses for educational and scientific test, and developing countries may wish to consider making greater use of these concessions.

**Ancillary Proprietary Regimes**

***Trade Secrets***

In modern economies trade secret law regulates the pace of competition by endowing second comers with an absolute right to reverse-engineer. To operate successfully under such a regime, developing countries must realign the concept of "transfer of technology" with the nature of competition on open markets. Technology is transferred through self-help methods of reverse engineering. The potential benefits of reverse-engineering unpatented technologies increase when advanced technologies are involved, notably biogenetic engineering, computer programmes and computer-aided design. The unpatented, non-copyrightable know-how underlying these technologies is often embodied in tangible products available to the public, which renders classical trade secret protection of doubtful efficacy. By ignoring this problem, the TRIPS Agreement provides entrepreneurs in developing countries with major opportunities, notwithstanding the extension of trade secret law under TRIPS, provided they are willing and able to master the art of reverse-engineering.

### Other Proprietary Regimes

The TRIPS Agreement mandates intellectual property protection for industrial designs, plant varieties and integrated circuit designs. Although the developed countries enjoy a clear advantage in advanced sectors of industrial design, more traditional sectors rooted in aesthetic appeal rather than technical efficiency remain accessible to firms in developing countries.

### Need for Multilateral Policies

Global economic integration increasingly requires that intangible creations receive minimum international standards of legal protection. Purely territorial intellectual property rights will thus give way to international sovereignty. However, the norms of that law represent a delicate balance between the interests of States at different stages of development, so that the evolution of international intellectual property law will have to accommodate these norms and that balance.

Efforts to implement higher intellectual property standards will put increasing strains on competition law, which is not directly covered by the TRIPS Agreement. Identifying the parameters of healthy competition valid for all players in an integrated world market will become a pressing task for the international community in a post-TRIPS world. These issues will be complicated by the fact that innovators, users, and second-comers all have different stakes in fashioning the rules of unfair competition law, and their interests will increasingly vary more with their economic roles than with the geopolitical affiliations of their respective national States.

Competition law must become an integral part of international discussions of intellectual property rights, and there is a great need for multilateral cooperation to achieve a marketwide balance between incentives to create and reasonable opportunities to imitate and improve upon technological innovation. These discussions should lead to an internationally agreed framework for promoting a transfer of technology that is compatible with the drive for greater economic efficiency. To the extent that such cooperation succeeds, it will contribute a new perspective to the notion of fair competition that should strengthen the prospects of all participants in the global marketplace.

## 21

# Employment and Poverty Alleviation

Today the key socio-economic problem is large-scale unemployment. Spreading joblessness brings many other problems in its wake. It erodes national income and living standards, aggravating the already grindingly difficult job of promoting development and alleviating poverty. Joblessness also raises government budget deficits, increasing macro-economic instability while soaking up investment for productive capital expenditure, education, training and relief aid. And joblessness ruins lives and communities by depriving people of the dignity and satisfaction that comes with earning one's keep and making a contribution to the well-being of family and society.

Theories about how best to nurture development (and thus create jobs) have shifted considerably over the last decade. The state's role has evolved, in the minds of many, from being a source of relief for the problems of unemployment, poverty and underdevelopment, to being a fundamental cause of these problems through the distorting impact of its intervention on the market.

However, the more market-oriented philosophy that grew up during the 1990s has yet to provide convincing solutions in practice at least not on a grand scale and especially not in terms of job creation as the present jobless economic recovery demonstrates.

The weakness of the current recovery and past approaches to economic development can be traced to the failure to consider employment as the predominant means of promoting growth and alleviating poverty. In policy circles it has too long been an almost ignored priority.

Current trends thus bode poorly, particularly as unemployment rates soar. In light of the circumstances, we need to begin re-examining some of the fundamental questions if only to find out what has gone wrong with the answers.

**Minimum Wage?**

Let's begin with wages. With corporate restructuring in full force on a global scale, are low wage rates required to raise employment and maximize profits? A top manager of a multinational consumer electronics group certainly thinks so; he liknened the perfect factory to a ship "so that we could move it around the world to where labour was cheapest". Perhaps, but this bottom-line emphasis on unit labour costs ignores at least two other factors; namely, that higher wages can act as a screen to select more productive workers and that higher wages translate into better productivity via improved worker nutrition, increased consumption and a generally healthier quality of life.

If higher wages bring these benefits (and it is an open question) should government insist that there be a minimum wage rate? Neo-classical economists tend to respond "no", assuming that a higher wage rate puts money into the pockets of some low wage workers while forcing many others out of work because companies cannot afford to pay them.

**Technology Transfer**

The impact of technology is another area in need of study. Technological innovation is usually labour-saving and tends to originate in industrialised countries, moving towards developing countries like India, Pakistan where labour tends to be low cost and abundant. Would it therefore make sense to slow down or somehow restrict technology transfer, especially to development markets, in the interest of preserving employment?

The answer here is clearly—no. Historical evidence abundantly demonstrates that attempts to retard technological progress bring about greater poverty and lower growth. Technology, infact, is at the heart of the new endogenous growth theory which is very much in vogue among development economists today. Slowing down or inhibiting technology transfer would certainly dash many countries' development hopes and aggravate poverty. However, the relationship between technology development, employment and poverty alleviation is not without its complications.

In the 1980s, the buzzword among development specialists was "appropriate technology", i.e., small-scale and labour-intensive technologies that would increase productive output while allowing an equilibrium solution to be found such that the ratio of the productivity of labour to that of capital is proportional to their relative prices. The conditions for this "small is beautiful" approach to technology tended to be best met in agricultural production. However, where manufacturing industry is concerned, the small-is-beautiful approach foundered badly when the only viable technological alternatives proved to be highly capital-intensive.

### Development Gap

A wide gap has emerged between developing countries with an inward focus (which tend to be protectionist and pursue policies of import substitution) and those with an outward focus and a policy of pursuing export-led growth. Competing in international markets requires technology that is as good as or better than that found in advanced, industrialised nations. Small, therefore, is not beautiful in the global manufacturing economy where product standards are high and the elasticity of substitution between labour and capital is very limited.

The drive to obtain state-of-the-art technology thus leads to a policy conundrum: it is a pre-condition for success in manufactured exports, but the impulse to compete successfully in this most lucrative sector speeds up the transfer of technology from the developed to the developing world, thus reinforcing the bias towards labour saving equipment in developing countries and accelerating a process that is seen as a source of job loss in the industrialised countries.

**Technology and Jobs**

Before concluding that modern technology transfer is inimical to employment in developing countries, we have to distinguish clearly between technology's static and dynamic consequences. In a static sense, it is true that highly capital-intensive export industries may not create much employment on a net basis, but the dynamic effects of technology transfer do contribute to economic growth. And growth, in turn, generates multiplier effects in the form of demand, which stimulates ancillary production activities (like food processing or consumer goods) that rely on more labour-intensive technologies.

The problem is that the diffusion and application of technology on a global scale blurs the categories of international product specialisation and creates a much more competitive and conflict-prone international environment.

For example, we have already seen the Asian Tigers move from producing goods such as textiles and processed food to producing hi-tech and value-added consumer durables. This advance is only possible due to the growth of human capital (facilitated by investment and higher incomes) and it leaves production of textiles to other industrialising countries, like Indonesia, the Philippines and now China. But the dynamic comes at the expense of jobs in industrialised regions, like the US and the EC, which lost more than a quarter of their work force in textiles during the 1980s. In spite of job losses, advanced countries continue to produce textiles, notwithstanding major differences in the hourly wage rates for spinning and weaving and the fact that essentially the same hi-tech equipment is being used in most production centres.

**Protectionism**

What has happened in textiles is happening in other industrial sectors (automobiles, for example) as well. The intense market competition is proving to be a source of trade conflicts, and possibly protectionism, as jobs come under increasing pressure.

For many workers and managers, the benefits of foreign direct investment look increasingly like a zero-sum game for employment, and there is a real risk that the tenuous link between overall growth and employment will break down altogether. It is hardly surprising that we are already seeing negatively affected workers and local businesses clamouring for protection in advanced countries.

**Governments role**

The concerned governments are suppose to carry out much of this research. The three initial lines of inquiry follow from three reasonable assumptions about the future.

- First, increase in welfare and consumption subsidies are out; investments in training and human capital are in. How can investments in human capital be directed to positive employment effects? Is it perhaps not time to explore more fully benefit schemes targeting the unemployed and the unskilled poor providing them with the type of subsidies that would enhance their human capital, improve their health and productivity through better nutrition and preventive medicine, and restore the dignity of holding a job?
- Second, given the quasi-inevitability of increased automation in manufacturing, how can other sectors (particularly agriculture and services) be developed to export their long-term potential for employment creation?
- Third, given the inevitable pressures of work and productivity in the global economy, what sort of alternative institutional arrangements need to evolve with respect to industrial relations, employment and work conditions?

Finding answers to these and other questions will require no small amount of new thinking, but parochialism or a failure of imagination would be fatal flaws in this global era.

# The Dynamics of Rural Poverty in India

Poverty is homogeneous only when considered from the point of view of income or consumption: the uniformity of the poor as a category exists only on the level of the fact that they have little to consume. When considered from the point of view of production, i.e., the circumstances in which the poor must operate to gain their income, the conditions of poverty are extraordinary diverse. A concrete grasp of these diverse circumstances is the first step in developing relevant instruments to address not only the problems of the poor, but also the challenge of taking advantage of the opportunities available to them.

The conventional means of measuring economic progress, such as Gross National Product per capita, tell us little about the real nature of poverty. In recent years this sort of yardstick has been supplemented by measurements of food security, income distribution, and social development (encompassing health and education). These offer the possibility of composite indices, allowing the development of more rounded characterisations and comparisons of poverty at the national level. However, these principally refer to the symptoms of poverty, not to the relational factors generating it. Poverty is not a state of being, it is the effect of dynamic processes. While it is important to know where poverty is greatest, it is critical to know why it exists. This inquiry necessarily leads away from the nature of the poor as individuals to the nature of their social and physical environment. Poverty is not only a personal phenomenon, it is a social status. As such, while its effects can be measured on the level of the individual, its causes must be sought elsewhere. From the point of view of poverty alleviation the process of becoming is just as important as the state of being.

At the heart of poverty is the inadequate access of the poor to productive resources. Low incomes tend to reflect inadequate means of production, not incompetent producers. However, poverty in India is not simply a reflection of private resources. A broad range of "external" factors impinge on incomes, among them the following:

### National Policies

One of the ironies of Indian development is that while no government wants poverty, many policies contribute to it—what is given in anti-poverty programmes is drained away by other policies. The poor do not always come out ahead in the balance—they are often net "donors" to the rest of society. Frequent reference is made to unsustainable forms of development—to urban over-expansion, industrialisation based on subsidies, and to public sector engorgement. What is less frequently realised is that the bill for these phenomena is often presented to the rural poor. Taxation of exports to sustain sectors with little export potential of their own and subsidised food imports to supply the urban population are policies that are often paid for by the rural poor. In many areas of India, exports are agricultural goods produced by small farmers. Here export taxes contribute to rural poverty. The same is true of "cheap" food imports which depress the prices paid to small farmers for their food crops.

"Structural imbalance" is not only a recipe for increasing external indebtedness, it is also a recipe for increasing the poverty of the rural population. The political weakness of the poor in most areas is not only the basis for inadequate poverty alleviation programmes and policies—it is the basis for an actual transfer of their income to more socially influential groups. While it is often correctly asserted that the poor are the first to suffer from adjustments involving public social expenditure cuts, it is often the case that they also have the most to gain from the elimination of policy-based economic distortions that reflect social power rather than productive efficiency and potential.

### Demographic Factors

Accelerated population growth is a long-term contributor to poverty. In India the incomes of the poor have declined, mortality rates are also falling, pushing the numbers up. In the meantime, land is becoming scarcer, plots more fragmented and the soil and pasture increasingly degraded. This phenomenon is not without its policy dimensions. As long as the poor remain undercapitalised, and essential determinant of household income is the amount of labour available to its household economic strategies favour large families. While population policy has a role to play, possibly more critical is a change in the economic environment. Access to capital and more secure income changes perceptions of the need for labour. In the medium and long-term, population dynamics are driven by the underlying productive systems. As long as the production systems of the poor remain underdeveloped, population growth remains high, restricting even the future possibility of development.

### Natural Resource Management and the Environment

If poverty is both cause and effect of rapid population expansion, so poverty is both cause and effect of many dimensions of degradation of the environment. Many of the rural poor, but by no means all, live in areas of extreme environmental fragility, a circumstance often prompted by high level of control by the better-off over more stable and productive resource areas. Here the poor are extraordinarily exposed to the dangers of erosion, whittling away at an already meager productive base. The threat is not entirely due to nature. Rather, poverty accelerates erosion. Without capital, the poor are frequently unable to invest in even traditional methods of soil and water conservation. And without sufficient land they are forced to shorten fallow periods, putting further strain on the resource base. As in the case of population growth, the result is strain not only on the poor, but on the entire Indian economy. Given the extremely limited economic alternatives, the solution to this problem is not to forbid the use of environmentally fragile resources to the poor, it is to change the conditions under which their use takes place. Access to conservation technology is important; but more so are security of land tenure and resources to invest.

Combating poverty means not only increasing the production of the poor, but also preserving and enhancing the long-term value of the resource they control. What this very often means, in practice is assisting the poor in reestablishing a stable relationship with fragile resource. Prevailing processes in many areas involve the gradual—and sometimes not so gradual—depletion of natural resources, to the detriment of all. Part of the answer to this is conservation. Part of the answer is also to provide viable economic alternatives to the poor, reducing their dependence on erosion-prone crop and livestock practices.

### Exploitative Intermediates

The poor are not unaware of the pressure upon them, and also of means of overcoming them. Their ability to respond, however, is severely impaired by social powerlessness. The poor are surrounded by a dense network of public and private factors reducing their freedom of action, and actually draining what few resources they do have. Members of the network include traders and moneylenders capitalising upon the economic weakness of the poor, and engaging them in unequal exchanges. They also include public agencies either indifferent to the requirements of the socially uninfluential, or actively engaged in extracting "surplus" for use by other groups. Not to be excluded from this are organisations which are ostensibly "for" the poor, but which, in fact, serve as systems of containment and control

# The WTO Dispute Settlement Mechanism

The Uruguay Round's new dispute settlement mechanism represents the new teeth of the World Trade Organisation (WTO). "The dispute settlement system of the WTO is a central element in providing security and predictability to the multilateral trading system", states the Understanding on Rules and Procedures Governing the Settlement of Disputes.

In the Final Act, WTO members have committed themselves not to take unilateral action against perceived violations of the trade rules. Instead, they have pledged to seek recourse in the new dispute-settlement system, and abide by its rules and procedures.

The Understanding emphasizes that prompt settlement of dispute is essential to the effective functioning of the WTO. Thus, it sets out in great detail the procedures and the timetable to be followed in resolving disputes—in contrast with the current GATT whose dispute-settlement provisions are contained in just two Articles. The existing GATT procedures have been built up over time through the evolution of customary practice, and later codified in decisions by GATT contracting parties—notably the 1979 Understanding and a provisional streamlining of the system in the 1989 Improvements following the Mid-term Review of the Round.

Under the WTO, there will be one *Dispute Settlement Body(DSB)* dealing with disputes arising from any agreement contained in the Final Act. Thus, the DSB will have the sole authority to establish panels, adopt panel and appellate reports, maintain surveillance of implementation of rulings and recommendations, and authorise retaliatory measures in cases of non-implementation of recommendations. This is a significant improvement over the current GATT, under which dispute settlement is fragmented between the Council and the various Tokyo Round Committees.

Other important new features distinguish the WTO mechanism from that of GATT: In the WTO, there has to be a consensus against the establishment of panels or adoption of panel reports for these decisions not to be made whereas the reverse is true for the current system. Thus, parties to the dispute in the new system can no longer block these decisions. Another new feature is the possibility of appealing panel decisions to a standing Appellate Body. And, in line with the new integrated nature of the WTO mechanism, complainants, as a last resort, may take retaliatory action—suspend concessions—under an agreement different from the one covering the dispute against a member that has not implemented adopted panel recommendations.

The following are the various stages involved in setting disputes in the WTO:

### Consultations

The aim of the WTO dispute-settlement mechanism is "to secure a positive solution to a dispute". Thus, developing a mutually acceptable solution consistent with WTO provisions to a problem between members is encouraged throughout the dispute-settlement process.

The first stage of settling disputes is the holding of consultations between the members concerned. Any member should reply promptly (within 10 days) to a request for consultations, and enter into consultations within 30 days from the date of the request. To ensure transparency, any request for consultations should be notified to the DSB in writing, providing the reasons for the request, including identification of the measure at issuc and the legal basis for the complaint.

If consultations fail, and if both parties so agree, the case at this stage can be brought to the WTO Director-General, who, acting in an ex-officio capacity, will be ready to offer good offices, conciliation or mediation to settle the dispute.

**Establishment of Panels**

If the member concerned do not respond to a request for consultations within 10 days or if the consultations fail to arrive at a solution after 60 days, the complainant can ask the DSB to establish a panel to examine the case.

The establishment of a panel is almost automatic. The procedures require that the DSB should establish a panel not later than the second time it considers the panel request, unless there is a consensus against the decision. This means that the government which is the subject of the complaint cannot block the establishment of the panel.

The determination of the panel's terms of reference as well as its composition is also straightforward. The Understanding provides for standard terms of reference that mandate the panel to examine the complaint in the light of the agreement cited, and to make findings that will assist the DSB in making recommendations or in giving rulings provided for in that agreement. The panel may operate under different terms of reference, if the parties concerned so agree.

The panel is to be constituted within 30 days of its establishment. The WTO Secretariat will suggest the names of three potential panellists to the parties to the dispute, drawing as necessary on a list of qualified persons (including, for example, those who have previously participated in panel proceedings, or have been representatives to GATT, or have taught international trade law). If the parties cannot agree on the panellists within 20 days from the establishment of the panel, at the request of either party, the Director-General, in consultations with the DSB Chairman and the Chairman of the relevant Committee or Council, will appoint the panellists. The panellists will serve in their individual capacities and will not be subject to government instructions.

### Panel Procedures

The understanding provides that the period in which the panel conducts its examination of the case—that is, from the time the terms of reference and composition of the panel are agreed to the time the panel's final report is given to the parties to the dispute—should not exceed six months. In cases of urgency, those relating to perishable goods, the timeframe is shortened to three months. In no case should the period from the establishment of the panel to the circulation of the report to the Members exceed nine months.

Detailed working procedures for the panel are set out in the Understanding (see chart).

### Adoption of Panel Reports

The WTO procedures provide that a panel report is to be adopted by the DSB within 60 days of issuance, unless one party notifies its decision to appeal or a consensus emerges against the adoption of the report.

The DSB cannot consider the adoption of a panel report earlier than 20 days after it has been circulated to members. Members who have objections to the report are required to state their reasons in writing for circulation before the DSB meeting at which the panel report will be considered.

### Appellate Review

A new feature of the WTO dispute settlement mechanism gives the possibility of appeal to either party in a panel proceeding. However, any appeal shall be limited to issues of law covered in the panel report and the legal interpretation developed by the panel.

All appeals will be heard by a standing Appellate body to be established by the DSB. This Appellate body will be composed of seven persons—broadly representative of the WTO membership—who will serve four-year terms. They are to be persons of recognised standing in the field of law and international trade, and not affiliated with any government.

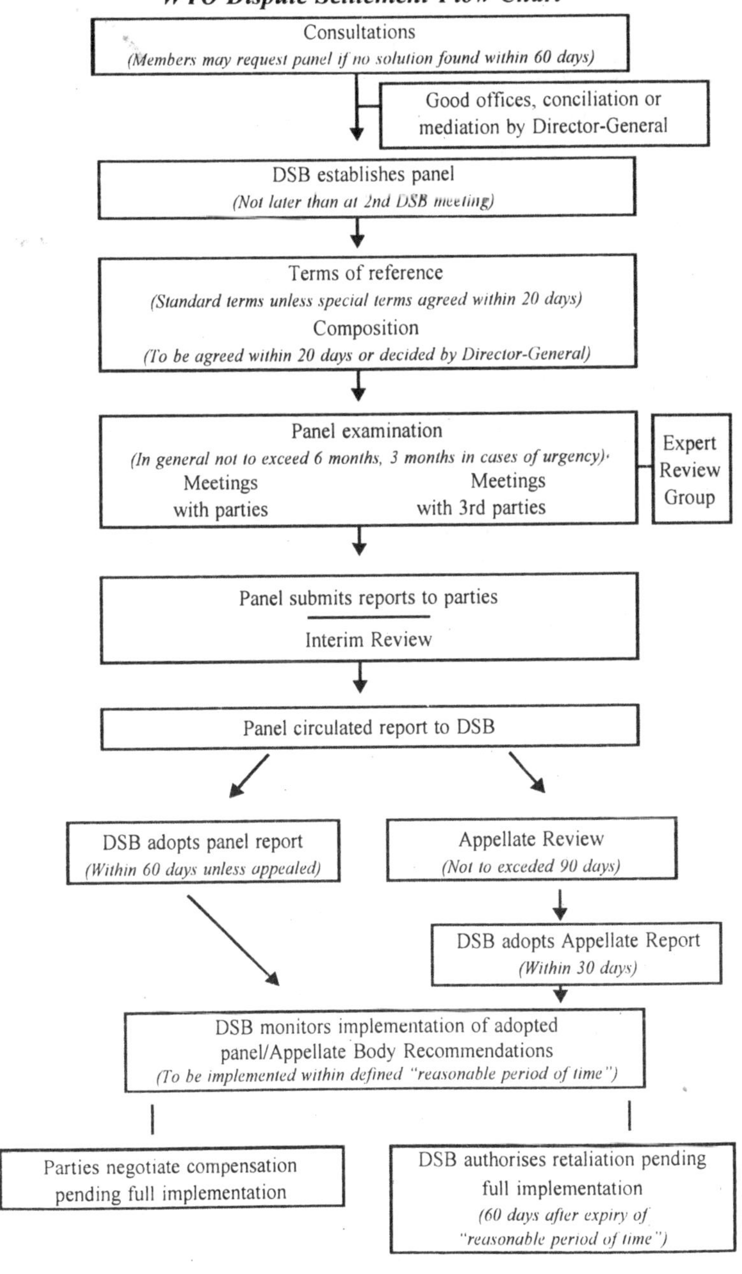
WTO Dispute Settlement Flow Chart
Consultations
(Members may request panel if no solution found within 60 days)
Good offices, conciliation or mediation by Director-General
DSB establishes panel
(Not later than at 2nd DSB meeting)
Terms of reference
(Standard terms unless special terms agreed within 20 days)
Composition
(To be agreed within 20 days or decided by Director-General)
Panel examination
(In general not to exceed 6 months, 3 months in cases of urgency)
Meetings with parties
Meetings with 3rd parties
Expert Review Group
Panel submits reports to parties
Interim Review
Panel circulated report to DSB
DSB adopts panel report
(Within 60 days unless appealed)
Appellate Review
(Not to exceded 90 days)
DSB adopts Appellate Report
(Within 30 days)
DSB monitors implementation of adopted panel/Appellate Body Recommendations
(To be implemented within defined "reasonable period of time")
Parties negotiate compensation pending full implementation
DSB authorises retaliation pending full implementation
(60 days after expiry of "reasonable period of time")

Three members of the Appellate body sit at any one time to hear appeals. They can uphold, modify or reverse the legal findings and conclusions of the panel. As a general rule, the appeal proceedings are not to exceed 60 days but in no case shall they exceed 90 days.

Thirty days after issuance, the Appellate body report is to be adopted by the DSB and unconditionally accepted by the parties to the dispute-unless there is, consensus against its adoption.

**Implementation**

The Understanding stresses that "prompt compliance with recommendations or rulings of the DSB is essential in order to ensure effective resolution of disputes to the benefit of all members."

At a DSB meeting held within 30 days of the adoption of the panel or appellate report, the party concerned must state its intentions in respect of the implementation of the recommendations. If it is impractical to comply immediately, the member will be given a "reasonable period of time" –to be set by the DSB—to do so. If it fails to act within this period, it is obliged to enter into negotiations with the complainant in order to determine a mutually acceptable compensation.

If after 20 days, no satisfactory compensation is agreed, the complainant may request authorisation from the DSB to suspend concessions or obligations against the other party. The procedures provide that the DSB should grant this authorisation within 30 days of the expiry of the "reasonable period of time" unless there is a consensus against the request.

If the member concerned objects to the level of suspension, the matter will be referred to arbitration. This will be carried out by the original panel members, and if this is not possible, by an arbitrator appointed by the WTO Director-General. Arbitration should be completed within 60 days of the expiry of the "reasonable period of time", and the resulting decision should be accepted by the parties concerned as final and not subject to another arbitration. The DSB, upon request, then authorises the suspension of concessions consistent with the findings of the arbitrator, unless there is a consensus to reject the request.

In principle, concessions should be suspended in the same sector as that in issue in the panel case. If this is not practicable or effective, the suspension can be made in a different sector of the same agreement. In turn, if this is not effective or practicable and if the circumstances are serious enough, the suspension of concessions may be made under another agreement.

In any case, the DSB will keep under surveillance the implementation of adopted recommendations or rulings, and any outstanding case will remain on its agenda until the issue is resolved.

# Safety First!

Throughout history, the violent side of nature has manifested itself in destructive phenomena such as floods, volcanic eruptions, severe storms, wildfires, earthquakes and tidal waves. Disasters and risks are part of our life, and they will continue to threaten, kill and destroy. "Zero risk" is out of reach in the contemporary world. The basic problem is how to prevent hazards from causing increasingly large-scale disasters. The answer is that the disastrous effects of natural phenomena will only be eliminated, reduced or stabilised when people decide to make cities, settlements, infrastructures and houses safe.

**A Culture of Prevention**

For people are the agents of disaster. "It's not the bullet that kills, it's the hole". Earthquakes and windstorms do not kill, the collapse of houses and buildings from shaking is the main cause of death. Natural hazards themselves are not on the increase; nor are they likely to be in the future. It is the frequency of natural disasters that is expected to grow, as well as their complexity, scope, gravity and destructive capacity. There will be an increase in multiple or synergistic-type disasters causing society-wide impacts. In a time of globalisation, large-scale damage caused by an earthquake in a world financial centre is bound to have an effect even on the economies of faraway countries.

Natural disasters are not always entirely "natural". On the one hand, natural forces are at work on planet whose environment is being altered day after day by humankind: floods are made moreover by deforestation, global warming more preoccupying by the unchecked emission of greenhouse gases. On the other, natural disasters will increasingly generate or magnify concurrent technological disasters. Floods can devastate chemical complexes, earthquakes can affect critical plants.

The good news is that disaster reduction is both possible and feasible. While we cannot prevent an earthquake or a windstorm from occurring, or a volcano from erupting, we can use the scientific knowledge and technical know-how that we already have in order to increase the earthquake and wind-resistance of houses and bridges, and to issue and disseminate early warnings of volcanic eruptions and organise proper community response to such warnings. The extent to which society puts this knowledge to effective use depends upon its social, cultural, political, economic, and even religious specificities.

**Informing the Public**

Disaster prevention and preparedness start with improving our understanding of risks by assessing the distribution in time and space and the intensity of the natural phenomena involved and the exposure of people and structures to them. On the basis of this assessment, protective measures may be taken such as land-use restrictions, adequate construction measures and wise environmental management. Detection and warning systems may be installed, and contingency and emergency plans be set up. One permanent measure of paramount importance is the education and information of the public.

A number of cases show that loss of life, injuries and physical damage can all be significantly reduced by the application of better warning and disaster prevention measures. Because of inadequate use of, and response to, warning, more than 300,000 people died in Bangladesh due to a cyclone in November 1970. In May 1985, better prediction and proper response to warning of a cyclone of the same intensity kept the death toll below 10,000. Similarly, appropriate warning and evacuation saved the people in India in various cyclones.

Disaster prevention measures cost much less than relief and reconstruction expenditure following a disaster, yet many decision-makers tend to focus on relief and to treat disaster situations in an ad hoc way when they are presented with them. Today most typical strategies are crisis-oriented. Furthermore, information about natural hazards and disaster reduction techniques is not well disseminated, and planners, project managers and communities do not integrate hazard management into development planning. Resources spent on relief and recovery continue to account for 96 per cent of all resources spent on disaster-related activities annually, leaving a pitiful 4 per cent for disaster prevention. It is high time to make a shift in emphasis from post-disaster reaction to pre-disaster action.

# The Dematerialisation of the World Economy

The first Industrial Revolution marked the transition from robber-and-plunder colonialism to the systematic development of the "overseas" territories in the framework of an international division of labour between raw materials suppliers and manufacturers of finished goods. There was a "historic integration" of the colonised areas in the development of their parent-states. What will the third Industrial Revolution do for the Third World? Will it now come to a "historic separation" ?

The end of the East-West conflict was reason enough to talk about a radical change in world politics. But at the same time an upheaval in the world economy is taking place that possibly will have even wider impacts. As a reference point for the following thoughts, three dimensions of this change are pointed out:

1. The upgrading of processing information rather than materials as object of economic activity (technological dimension) ;

2. The evolvement of global communications networks (sociocultural dimension) ;

3. The change of the nature of work (socio-economic dimension).

All three dimensions can be summarised under the buzzphrase "tertialisation of the world economy."

In that respect, talk of the "Third Industrial Revolution" is misleading. It is not about a third epoch of industrialisation, but about the beginning of a de-industrialisation, the transition from the industrial to the information society.

**Historic Separation?**

In the 1960s and early 1970s, there was often talk of the Third World as the Third Sector of the world economy. Also then the Third World was not much more than an "imaginary community". But as such it had a certain significance in world politics. This implied not only its strategic role in the East-West conflict and its ideological function as the supporter of different "third paths" between capitalism and socialism. It was also about the Third World's attested "chaos power". That linked the fear (in the North) and the hope (in the South) that the developing countries would be in a position to cut off the industrial nations from supplies of important raw materials, thus putting them under pressure. But it was soon seen that both sides had over estimated this possibility, even with regard to oil. Instead of supply bottlenecks arising, raw materials prices plummeted. For some commodities, the fall in prices exceeded those of the Great Depression of 1929/30.

This was due, inter alia, to the conjunction of lower demand from the industrial nations and expansion of production by the raw materials suppliers. Business activities dependent upon the supply of raw materials are tending to lose importance compared with the overall development of the global economy. The reason for this is to be seen in the transition from a material to an information economy.

This transition is taking place in line with the revolutionising of data transmission and the expansion of financial transactions which are not directly related to changes in the production of materials. The speed of the changes is remarkable.

However, the dematerialisation of business activities does not lead to decoupling of the Third World from the world economy. Declining market shares in world trade are not the expression of separation, but a loss of the affected countries positions in the world economy. Thus, the impact of dematerialisation is "only" that the negotiating positions of raw materials suppliers vis-a-vis the industrial nations will deteriorate further.

**Differentiation of the Third World**

But the radical change in the global economy is affecting some developing countries worse than others. Sub-saharan Africa, and some countries in West and South Asia and Latin America are being pushed back further. The oil-producing countries with their high per capita export earnings will be able to hold their positions in the world economy for some time to come. The threshold countries of East and South-East Asia can expand theirs so long as they can continue to attract a growing share of global industrial production, and at the same time participate in the tertialisation of the world economy in the shape of rapidly-growing financial transactions. Thereby it should be noted that the degree of tertialisation in itself is not an adequate indicator for economic avant-gardism. Brazil exhibits a high degree of tertialisation in combination with a low macroeconomic development dynamics. A good part of its tertialisation is being achieved by speculative financial transactions with their inherently greater risks and uncertainties that in the industrial countries. Such dangers have been demonstrated by Mexico's peso crisis and its repercussions on the whole of Latin America.

In some Third World countries, a "location annuity" has replaced the old raw materials one. Here it's about providing locations for off-shore transactions which offer international capital traders a maximum freedom of movement combined with low taxation. Suitable for such operations are small countries which, despite low levy rates, achieve significant income in macroeconomic terms.

The radical changes in the world economy are spurring the differentiation of the Third World without, however, necessarily fostering a dissolution of the Third World as an "imaginary community". It is precisely the advanced countries of East and South-East Asia that are showing a certain interest in the formulation of joint positions of the "South" in order to secure their own positional gains in the global economy. It's not by chance that the non-aligned countries and the Group of 77 have formed a joint coordination committee, and that the ASEAN countries are changing course on the international human rights policy.

Hitherto, the developing countries' strategy was to broaden the concept of human rights as a justification for demands on the industrial nations. But of late some developing countries, led by the ASEAN states, have questioned the universal validity of human rights even after their universality was confirmed by consensus at the Conference on Human Rights in Vienna in 1993. Playing a role in this policy is the governments' fear that due to the expansion of global communications networks, the behaviour patterns and preferences of their own people could in some way become similar to those of the West. As the rulers see it, that would be detrimental to the continuation of the development models practised so far.

### Internet Creates New Cultural Dimension

Much information which Asian governments view as subversive in already globally available on the Internet. The old struggle over the world information order, which at first was primarily a clinch between East and West, is thus taking on a new dimension. For with the growing importance of computer literacy to a country's ability to assert itself on world markets, the Asian threshold countries have not only an interest in controlling the on-line communication but also to expand it and the know-how that it requires.

Even the critics of any interventions in the internet and other global communications networks must admit that modern communications technologies are politically blind and their use in itself does not represent progress. The setting up and expansion of global information highways will offer forum not only to people who want to use it for education and enlightenment, but also to all shades of fundamentalists. These highways will not necessarily bring the misery of many

Third World regions closer to the industrial countries, but possibly rather strengthen the tendency to process all world events as entertainment.

**Global Two-thirds Society**

The gravest aspect of the current upheaval in the world economy is its negative impact on jobs. The information economy needs for fewer workers than an economy based on materials. Instead, the demands on the skills of the workers are growing. Twenty per cent of the world workforce will in future be employed as (overworked) "intelligence workers". Eighty per cent will work part-time, if they are not underemployed or jobless. So the tertialisation of the global economy delivers more underemployment rather than more leisure time. The workers who are rationalised out of their jobs in the industrial sector cannot be absorbed by the service sector because it, too, is not left untouched by rationalisation measures. The civil service is also cutting back on staff. At all levels, there's a race to make the greatest possible savings on payrolls. At the same time, there's growing pressure to cut costs in providing for the victims of this development. That means thinning out the social security safety net.

The bottom line is that the two-thirds society, which developmental action groups hitherto assumed was limited to the Third World, is spreading worldwide. That, however, will not in the foreseeable future lead to an amendment of the North-South disparities. It's true that the change in the global economy is taking place faster, and to a greater extent in the industrial nations. But rationalisation is also happening in the developing countries in a bid to boost their competitiveness. So the upheaval in the world economy aggravates the problems which exist in a majority of the developing countries, while creating new ones in the industrial nations. The need for action on the North-South policy is growing, while the industrial nations' scope for concessions and compromises is shrinking. The new social question which is now crystallising at global level is not being answered. The consequences are unforeseeable.

**Another Loser?**

It's more probable that a sharpening of the North-South confrontation is to be reckoned with. For the industrial nations will attempt to keep the social costs of the information economy at bay for as long as possible. The trade unions will thereby compete with the developing countries for jobs for their members. But this policy has its limits precisely because of the peaking of the problems in the industrial nations. Overstepping these limits means war, and passively accepting them chaos and social decay. Solutions could be sought in two directions: effective taxation of the information economies, and the creation of jobs in the non-profit sector. But it's possible there are no global solutions for global problems. That would mean for at least part of the Third World a renewal of the old debate on partial decoupling from the world economy.

# 26

# Economics and Sustainable Development

Economists and ecologists were once seen as enemies: environmental protection, it was thought, could only be achieved at the expense of economic growth. The misconception persists at the extremes among both the most fundamentalist Greens and the most ideological free marketers. But increasingly it is now being recognised the development and care for the environment go hand in hand. This interdependence is coalescing in the new and necessary discipline of environmental economics.

Conventional economic patterns have often assumed that growth and technical progress will nullify all resource an environmental limits. Environmental economics recognises that the world's natural capital underpins all development, and that it is rapidly becoming scarcer as human demands exceed the globe's long-term carrying capacity. Government of India has introduced environmental measures over the last two decades, but need to move further towards integrating them into economic policies. There can be no real sustainable development unless environment and development policies are integrated at the very beginning of the decision-making process.

## Quantifying the Environmental Cost

One of the first steps is to work out the true costs of polluting and depleting the world's natural resources, such as its soil, air and water, the climate and the ozone layer. These have often been regarded as free goods, and it was believed that the world has an infinite capacity to absorb the effects of human activities. Environmental economists, recognising that the social and economic costs of degradation are very great, are trying to quantify them. They say that this will make possible better use of such tools as cost-benefit analysis, environmental impact assessment and risk assessment, and the production of national income accounts which reflect the depletion and degradation of natural resources. As these costs are identified and quantified, economic policy can increasingly be developed with sustainable development as the primary objective. Achieving sustainable development requires industrialised and developing countries to make dramatic changes in national and international policies based on a global partnership. The greenhouse effect, the destruction of the ozone layer, the extinction of species and contamination of the oceans and other environmental problems affect us all, no matter which corner of the globe we inhabit.

The first and essential step in overcoming a difficulty is to recognise it and understand it. Concern over the difficulties related to sustainability has led scientists and national and international institutions to study the concept and suggest ways of meeting its many requirements. Indicators have been established to measure pollution levels, soil erosion, salinisation, deforestation an a host of environmental problems. Evaluating the impact of such natural resource-use on ecosystems is a major step towards finding the necessary solutions.

For example, it has become clear, on a macroeconomic level, that national accounting systems fail to reflect these effects adequately. Deterioration of the world's rivers, land degradation, air pollution and contamination of the seas are not taken into consideration. Inadequate accounting distorts reality and gives a false idea of the consequences of growth and production.

On a microeconomic level, much is being done to redefine production costs. Incorporating the cost of waste management and internalising negative external impacts within production prices are beneficial aspects of the economics of sustainability.

Steps are being taken to evaluate public and commonly held assets and to put a price on them, even though they may not be subject to market forces. These are only in the earliest stage but they will allow for more accurate evaluation of the world's natural capital. Fiscal, market, quota and other instruments are being developed to enforce change in the way in which certain resources are used. Examples include markets for transferable emission quotas or compensatory taxation mechanisms designed to ensure that economic forces act to reduce greenhouse gas emissions. Efforts at impact analysis—and in a general sense, cost-benefit analysis—permit rough estimations of the impact that projects might have on ecosystems.

**Long-term Repercussions**

These instruments carry significant limitations but they are important nevertheless because they attempt to quantify impacts on the natural world and to achieve a more rational use of natural resources. The development of such instruments and evaluation techniques will have significant repercussions in the formulation of sustainable long-term policies. But we must bear in mind that sustainability is not just an economic issue: it is also a political and cultural one.

The concept of sustainability demands an alternative view point in which humankind and the natural world are perceived as a unit-as different yet mutually sustaining aspects of a whole. This perception is not incompatible with progress. It does not renounce development. It simply seeks to affirm life and refuses to discriminate between the means and the end.

It understands that happiness cannot be achieved by destructive means. The questions of how to produce and how to consume therefore become extremely important. Neither should be at the expense of the future or of the natural world. Efficiency is not limited to the links between investment, products and prices: it must address the rational use of resources, including environmental and cultural consequences, both in the long and the short-term.

Very considerable adjustments must be made in the interest of sustainable development. They demand a reassessment of all our activities which cannot, logically, be done overnight. It is a long and continuous process, characterised by steadfastness and compromise.

# Fertility Rates:

## *The Decline is Stalling*

During the 1970's, one of the population trends was the reduction in the total fertility rate in several key countries, including the world's two largest nations—China and India. (The fertility rate measures the average number of children born to women in their childbearing years.) In China the rate dropped precipitously from 6.4 children per woman in 1968 to 2.2 in 1980. In India the decline was more modest, but still significant: from 5.8 children per woman between 1966 and 1971 to 4.8 children between 1976 and 1981.

These trends helped slow the rate of world population growth from 2.1 per cent between 1965 and 1970 to 1.7 per cent between 1975 and 1980. At that point, however, the decline in the number of children that women were having in these two population giants stalled.

In China, despite the most aggressive and least democratic population control program in the world, the fertility rate remained around 2.5 throughout much of the 1980s as couples continued to want to marry young and to have two or more children. In India, the overzealous promotion of family planning by the ruling Congress Party through 1977 apparently backfired after the party's defeat and progress towards lower birth rates ran out of steam.

One important lesson from these experiences is that governments must do more than just supply contraceptives;

they need to lower the demand for children by making fundamental changes that improve women's lives and increase their access to and control over money, credit and other resources.

Many countries still register fertility rates above replacement level (See Table), which is generally 2.1 children per woman or basically two children per couple. The total fertility rate for the world as a whole in 1995 was 3.3, ranging from 1.8 in more developed nations to 4.4 in less developed ones (excluding China). In a number of countries, such as Brazil, Egypt, Indonesia, Mexico and Thailand, fertility rates have been dropping as they did in the 1970s in China and India. At the same time, developing countries have not yet entered the demographic transition.

The demographic transition occurs when both birth rates and death rates in a country drop from historically high levels to low ones that translate into a stable population – one that merely replaces itself with each new generation. Traditionally, although not always, death rates have declined first, following the spread of sanitation and improved healthcare overall. Rapid population growth often follows this first phase of the demographic transition, as the gap between fertility and mortality rates widens for a time. Eventually, however, fertility rates fall too.

As the moment, they remain high in a number of countries. The reasons include unequal rights and opportunities for women, as well as inadequate access to birth control. Whatever the reason, the effect is the same: 67 countries, home to 17 per cent of the world population, are at best in the early stages of a transition to low fertility rates. Most of them are in Africa and South Asia, and their population is likely to double in 20 to 25 years.

This is leading to a two-tiered demographic world that is every bit as worrying as the world of economic haves and have-nots. Countries such as Nigeria and Pakistan are finding it harder to keep up with the demand for food, healthcare, jobs, housing and education than countries that are in the middle of the demographic transition.

**Population Size, Fertility Rate and Doubling Time—20 Largest Countries, 1995**

| *Country* | *Fertility Population (millions)* | *Rate (average number of children per woman)* | *Doubling Time (years)* |
|---|---|---|---|
| Italy | 58 | 1.3 | 3466 |
| Germany | 81 | 1.4 | * |
| Japan | 125 | 1.5 | 217 |
| United Kingdom | 58 | 1.8 | 267 |
| France | 58 | 1.8 | 169 |
| Russia | 149 | 1.7 | 990 |
| United States | 258 | 2.0 | 92 |
| China | 1178 | 1.9 | 60 |
| Thailand | 57 | 2.4 | 49 |
| Indonesia | 188 | 3.0 | 42 |
| Brazil | 152 | 3.6 | 46 |
| Turkey | 61 | 3.6 | 32 |
| Mexico | 90 | 3.4 | 13 |
| India | 97 | 3.9 | 34 |
| Vietnam | 72 | 4.0 | 31 |
| Philippines | 5 | 4.1 | 28 |
| Egypt | 8 | 4.6 | 30 |
| Pakistan | 122 | 6.7 | 23 |
| Iran | 3 | 6.6 | 20 |
| Nigeria | 5 | 6.6 | 23 |

**Source:** Population Reference Bureau, 1995 World Population Data Sheet (Washington, DC. 1995).

Even when a country does reach replacement-level fertility, its population can continue growing for decades. There is a built-in momentum created by all the people who have yet to enter their childbearing years. Indeed, the decline in the world's population growth rate stalled in the 1980s in part because even in China, India and other countries where fertility rates had been dropping, large number of people who had been born in the 1960s reached childbearing age. So even if couples had two or three children instead of five or six, as their parents did, the population would grow substantially.

For the world as a whole, even if replacement–level fertility had been achieved in 1990, the population would continue to grow until it reached 8.4 billion in 2150 because of all the young people already alive. This built-in momentum obviously limits how quickly any country can stop population growth. Nevertheless, reaching replacement-level fertility is an all-important first step. The 67 countries that have not yet begun the demographic transition—nations in which invariably the government believes fertility levels are too high—could move in the right direction by providing the contraceptive and healthcare services that would help couples have only the number of children they desire.

# Bibliography


Agarwal, Bina. 1992. "Gender Relations and Food Security: Coping with Seasonality, Drought and Famine in South Asia." In Lourdes Beneria and Shelley Feldman, (eds) *Unequal Burden: Economic Crises, Persistent Poverty, and Women's Work*. Boulder, Colo.: Westview Press.

Agarwal, Bina. 1997. "Bargaining and Gender Relations: Within and Beyond the Household." *Feminist Economics* 3(1): 1-51.

Akerlof, George A., and Rachel E. Kranton. 1999 *Economics and Identity*. Washington, D.C.: Brookings Institute.

Alkire, Sabina. 1999. "Operationalizing Amartya Sen's Capability Approach to Human Development: A Framework for Identifying 'Valuable' Capabilities, "Ph. D. diss, Oxford University.

Baulch, Bob, 1996a. "Neglected Trade-Offs in Poverty Measurement." *IDS Bulletin* 27(1): 36-42.

Baulch, Bob, 1996b. "The New Poverty Agenda: A Disputed Consensus." *IDS Bulletin* 27(1): 1-10.

Bebbington A., and T. Perreault. 1999. "Social Capital, Development and Access to Resources in Highland Ecuador." *Economic Geography*. October.

Beneria, Lourdes. 1989. "Gender and the Global Economy." In Arthur MacEwan and William Tabb, eds. *Instability and Change in the Global Economy*. New York: Monthly Review Press.

Berelson, Bernard, 1954. "Content Analysis." *Handbook of Social Psychology*. Vol. 1. Reading, Mass.: Addison-Wesley.

Bhatt, Mihir. 1999. "Natural Disasters as National Shocks to the Poor and Development." Disaster Mitigation Institute, Ahmedabad, India.

Booth, David Jeremy Holland, Jesko Hentschel, Peter Lanjouw, and Alicia Herbert. 1998. *Participation and Combined Methods in African Poverty Assessment: Renewing the Agenda*. Department for International Development (DFID), U.K: Social Development Division and Africa Division.

Bradley, Christine. 1994 "Why Male Violence against Women is a Development Issue: Reflections from Papua New Guinea." In Miranda Davies, ed. *Women and Violence: Realities and Responses, Worldwide.* London: Zed Books.

Brunetti, Aymo, Gregory Kisunko, and Beatrice Weder. 1997. "Institutions in Transition" Reliability of Rules and Economic Performance in Former Socialist Countries." Policy Research Working Paper 1809 Washington, D.C.: World Bank.

Carvalho, Soniya, and Howard White. 1997. " Combining the Quantitative and Qualitative Approaches to Poverty Measurement and Analysis: The Practice and the Potential." Technical Paper 366. Washington, D.C.: World Bank.

Castellas, Manuel. 1997, *The Power of Identity.* Malden, Mass.: Blackwell Publishers.

Cernea, Michael 1979. "Entry Points for Sociological Knowledge in the Project Cycle." Agricultural and Rural Development Department. Washington, D.C.: World Bank.

Cernea, Michael, and Ayse Kudat. 1997. "Social Assessments for Better Development; Case Studies in Russia and Central Asia." Environmentally Sustainable Development Studies and Monograph Series 16. Washington, D.C.: World Bank.

Cernea, Michael, with the assistance of April Adams. 1994. "Sociology Anthropolgy and Development: An Annotated Bibliography of World Bank Publications 1975-1993." Environmentally and Sustainable Development Studies and Monograph Series 3. Washington, D.C.: World Bank.

Cernea, Michael. ed. 1985. *Putting People First.* New York; Oxford University Press.

Chambers, Robert. 1989. "Editorial Introduction: Vulnerability, Coping and Policy." *IDS Bulletin* 20: 1.

Chambers, Robert. 1994. "The Origins and Practice of Participatory Rural Appraisal." *World Development* 22(7). Washington, D.C.: World Bank.

Chambers, Robert. 1997. "Whose Reality Counts? Putting the First Last." London: Intermediate Technology Publications.

Chambliss, William J. 1999. *Power, Politics, and Crime.* Boulder, Colo.: Westview Press.

Charmes, Jacques. 1998. "Informal Sector, Poverty and Gender: A Review of Empirical Evidencee." Contributed paper for *World Development Report 2000.* Washington, D.C.: World Bank October.

Dahle, Cheryl. 1999. "Social Jusitice—Alan Khazei and Vanessa Kirsch." Fast Company, Issue 30, December 1999, www. fastcompany. Com.

Dasgupta, Partha, and Ismail Serageldin 1999. *Social Capital: A Multifaceted Perspective.* Washington, D.C.; World Bank.

Davies, Miranda, ed. 1994. *Women and Violence: Realities and Responses Worldwide.* London: Zed Books.

Dollar, David, and Roberta Gatti, 1995. "Gender Inequality, Income, and Growth Are: Good Times Good for Women?" Policy Research Report on Gender and Development, No. I. Wahington, D.C. World Bank.

Economist Intelligence Unit. 1997. *Armenia Country Profile, 1996-97.* London: The Economist Intelligence Unit, Ltd.

Edwards, Michael, and David Hulme, eds. 1992. *Making a Difference: NGOs and Development in a Changing World.* London: Earthscan Publications.

Edwards, Robert, and Michael W. Foley. 1997. "Social Capital and the Political Economy of Our Discontent." *American Behavioral Scientist,* 40(5). 669-78.

Esman, Milton J., and Norman Uphoff. 1984. *Local Organizations Intermediaries in Rural Development.* Ithaca, N.Y.: Cornell University Press.

Fajnzylber, Pablo, David Lederman, and Norman Loayza. 1998. *What Causes Violent Crime?* Office of the Chief Economist, Latin America and the Caribbean Region. Washington, D.C.: World Bank.

Floro, Maria Sagrario. 1995. "Economic Restructuring, Gender and the Allocation of Time." *World Development* 23: 1913-29. Washington, D.C.: World Bank.

Folbre, Nancy. 1991. "Women on Their Own: Global Patterns of Female Headship." In Rita S. Gallin, Anne Feguson, and Janice Harper, eds. *The Women and International Development Annual.* Vol. 4. Boulder, Colo.: Westview Press.

Foley, Michael W., and Robert Edwards. 1996. "The Paradox of Civil Society." *Journal of Democracy* 7(3): 38-52

Foster, James and Amartya Sen. 1997. "On Economic Inequality after a Quarter Century." 2nd ed. Oxford: Clarendon Press.

Fox, Jonathan. 1993. *The Politics of Food in Mexico: State Power and Social Mobilization.* Ithaca: Cornell University Press.

Galtung, Johan. 1994. *Human Rights in Another Key.* Cambridge, U.K.: Polity Press.

Gelles, Richard J., and Murray Straus 1998. *Intimate Violence.* New York: Simon and Schuster.

Giddens, Anthony. 1984. *The Constitution of Society.* Oxford: Blackwell.

Goetz, Anne Marie. 1998. "Women in Politics and Gender Equity on Policy: South Africa and Uganda." *Review of African Political Economy* 76: 241-62.

Greeley, Martin. 1994 "Measurement of Poverty and Poverty of Measurment." *IDS Bulletin 25*(2).

Grootaert, Christiaan, and Deepa Narayan. 1999. "Local Institutions, Poverty and Household Welfare in Bolivia." Social Development Family. Environmentally and Socially Sustainable Development Network. Washington, D.C.: World Bank.

Grootaert, Christiaan. 1998. "Social Capital: The Missing Link?" Social Capital Initiative Working Paper No. 3. Social Development Family. Washington, D.C.: World Bank.

Grootaert, Christiaan. 1999. "Social Capital, Household Welfare, and Poverty in Indonesia." Policy Research Working Paper 2148. Social Development Family., Washington, D.C.: World Bank.

Holland, Jeremy, and James Blackburn, eds. 1998. *Whose Voice? Participatory Research and Policy Change.* London: Intermediate Technology Publications.

Hyden, Goran. 1997. "Civil, Society, Social Capital, and Development: Dissection of a Complex Discourse." *Studies in Comparative International Development* 32:3-30.

Jackson, Cecile. 1996. "Rescuing Gender from the Poverty Trap." *World Development* 23:489-504.

Jain, Devaki. 1996. "Panchayat Raj: Women Changing Governance." Gender in Development Programme. United Nations Development Programme, New York.

Kabeer, Naila, and Ramya Subrahmanian. 1996. *Institutions, Relations and Outcomes: Framework and Tools for Gender-aware Planning.* University of Sussex; U.K.: Institute of Development Studies.

Kabeer, Naila. 1997. "Women, Wages and Intra-household Power Relations in Urban Bangladesh." *Development and Change 28* (2): 261-302.

Kaufmann, Georgia. 1997. "Watching the Developers: A Partial Ethnography." In R.D. Grillo and R.L. Stirrat, eds. *Discourses of Development: Anthroplogical Perspectives.* Oxford: Berg Press.

Korten, David C. 1990. *Getting to the 21st Century: Voluntary Action and the Global Agenda.* West Hartford, Conn.: Kumarian Press.

Krishan, Anirudh, Norman Uphoff, and Milton J. Esman (eds). 1997. *Reason for Hope: Instructive Experience in Rural Development.* West Hartford, Conn.: Kumarian Press.

Krishna, Anirudh, and Norman Uphoff. 1999. "Mapping and Measuring Social Capital: A Conceptual and Empirical Study of Collective Action for Conserving and Developing Watersheds in Rajasthan, India." Social Capital Initiative Working Paper No. 13. Washington, D.C.: World Bank.

Leach, Melissa, Robin Mearns, and Ian Scoones. 1997. *Community-Based Sustainable Development: Consensus or Conflict?* University of Sussex, U.K.: Institute of Development Studies.

Lipton, Michael, and Martin Ravallion. 1995. "Poverty and Policy." In Jere Richard Behrman and Thirukodikaval Nilakanta Srinivasan, eds. *Handbook of Development Economic.* Vol. 3. Amsterdam: Elsevier Press.

MacEwen Scott, Alison. 1995. "Informal Sector or Female Sector? Gender Bias in Urban Labor Maket Models." In Diane Elson, ed., *Male Bias in the Development Process.* 2nd ed. Manchester, U.K.: Manchester University Press.

Marshall, Gordon. 1994. *The Concise Oxford Dictionary of Sociology.* New York: Oxford University Press.

Max-Neef, Manfred. 1993. *Human Scale Development: Conception, Application, and Further Reflections.* London: Apex Press.

Milanovic, Branko. 1998. *Income, Inequality, and Poverty during the Transition from Planned to Market Economy.* Regional and Sectoral Studies. Washington, D.C.: World Bank.

Milimo, John T. 1995. "An Analysis of Qualitative Information on Agriculture: from Beneficiary Assessments, Participatory Poverty Assessments and Other studies which used Qualitative Research Methods." Ministry of Agriculture, Food, and Fisheries. Lusaka, Zambia.

Moore, Mick, and James Putzel. "Thinking Strategically about Politics and Poverty." IDS Working Paper 101. University of Sussex, U.K.: Institute of Development Studies.

Moser, Caroline, Annika Tornqvist, and Bernice van Bronkhorst. 1998."Mainstreaming Gender and Development in the World Bank: Progess and Recommendations." Washington, D.C.: World Bank.

Moser, Caroline. 1998. *The Asset-Vulnerability Framework: Reassessing Urban Poverty Reduction Strategies.* Washington, D.C.: World Bank.

Narayan, Deepa and Michael Cassidy. 1999. "A Dimensional Approach to Measuring Social Capital: Development and Validation of a Social Capital Inventory." Draft. Washington, D.C.: World Bank.

Narayan, Deepa, and Katrinka Ebbe. 1997. "Design of Social Funds: Participation, Demand Orientation, and Local Organizational Capacity." Discussion Paper No. 375. Washington, D.C. World Bank.

Narayan, Deepa, and Lant Pritchett. 1999. "Cents and Sociability: Household Income and Social Capital in Rual Tanzania." *Economic Development and Cultural Change* (47)4: 871-878

Narayan, Deepa, and Lyra Srinivasan. 1994. *Participatory Development Tool Kit: Training Materials for Agencies and Communities* Washington, D.C.: World Bank.

Narayan, Deepa, and Talat Shah. 2000. *Gender Inequity, Poverty, and Social Capital.* Research Report on Gender Development, Working Paper Series. Washington, D.C.: World Bank.

Narayan, Deepa. 1999. "Bonds and Bridges: Social Capital and Poverty." Policy Researvh Working Paper 2167. Policy Research Department. Washington, D.C.: World Bank.

North, Douglas. 1990. "Institutions and their Consequences for Economic Performance." In Karen Schweers Cook and Margaret Levi, eds. *The Limits of Rationality.* Chicago, Ill.: University of Chicago.

Norton Andy, and Thomas Stephens. 1995. "Participation in Poverty Assessments." Social Development Paper 9. Washington, D.C.: World Bank.

Orbach, Susie. 1999. "Psychoanalysis and Social Policy." Seminar paper presented to the World Bank, Washington, D.C., April.

Partes, Alejandro. 1998. "Social Capital: Its Origins and Applications in Modern Sociology." *Annual Review of Sociology* 22: 1-24.

Patton, Michael Quinn. 1990. *Qualitative Evaluation and Research Methods.* Newbury Park, Calif.: Sage Publications.

Pottier, Johan. 1997. "Towards an Ethnography of Participatory Appriaisal and Research." In R.D. Grillo and R.L. Stirrat, eds.

*Discourses of Development: Anthropological Perspectives.* Oxford, U.K.: Berg Press.

Putnam Robert, Robert Leonardi, and Raffaella Y. Nanetti. 1993. *Making Democracy Work: Civic Traditions in Modern Italy.* Princeton, N.J.: Princeton University Press.

Ravallion, Martin 1995. "China's Lagging Poor Areas." *American Economic Review, Papers and Procedures* 89: 301-5.

Ray, Raka, and Anna Kortweg. 1999. "Women's Movements in the Third World: Indentity, Mobilization and Autonomy." *Annual Review of Sociology 25:* 47-71.

Rietbergen-McCracken, Jennifer, and Deepa Narayan. 1998. "Participatory Tools and Techniques: A Resource Kit for Participation and Social Assessment" Social Policy and Resettlement Division, Environment Department. Washington, D.C.: World Bank.

Robb, Caroline. 1999. "Can the Poor Influence Poverty? Participatory Poverty Assessments in the Developing World." Washington, D.C.: World Bank.

Rodrik, Dani. 1998. "Globalization, Social Conflict and Economic Growth." *World Economy* 21(1): 43-58.

Rupesinhe, Kumar, and Marcial Rubio. 1994 *The Culture of Violence.* New York; United Nations University Press.

Salmen, Lawrence. 1987. *Listen to the People.* New York; Oxford University Press.

Salmen, Lawrence. 1995. "Participatory Poverty Assessment: Incorporating Poor People's Perpectives into Poverty Assessment Work." Social Development Paper No. 11 Washington , D.C.: World Bank.

Salmen, Lawrence. 1998. "Toward a Listening Bank; A Review of Best Practices and the Efficacy of Beneficiary Assessment." Social Development Paper No. 23.Washington, D.C.: World Bank.

Sartori, Giovanni. 1997. "Understanding Pluralism." *Journal of Democracy* 8(4): 58-69.

Schuler, Sidney Ruth, Syed M. Hashemi, and Shamsul Huda Badal. 1998. "Men's Violence against Women in Rural Bangladesh: Undermined or Exacerbated by Microcredit Programmes?" *Development in Practice* 8 (2): 148-57.

Schwartz, S.H. 1994. "Are There Universal Aspects in the Structure and Contents of Human Values?" *Journal of Social Issues* 50(4): 19-45.

Sen, Amartya K. 1981. *Poverty and Famines.* Oxford: Clarendon Press.

Sen, Amartya K. 1983. "Poor, Relatively Speaking." *Oxford Economic Papers* 35: 153-69. Reprinted in *Resources, Values and Development.*

Sen, Amartya K. 1984. "Rights and Capabilities." In Amartya K. Sen, ed., *Resource, Values and Development.* Oxford, U.K.: Blackwell.

Sen, Amartya K. 1985. "A Sociological Approach to the Measurement of Poverty: A Reply to Professor Peter Townsend." *Oxford Economic Papers* 37; 669-76.

Sen, Amartya K. 1992. *Inequality Reexamined.* Cambridge, Mass; Harvard University Press.

Sen, Amartya K. 1993. "Economic Regress: Concepts and Features." *Proceedings of the World Bank Annual Conference on Development Economics,* 315-54.

Sen, Amartya K. 1997. *On Economic Inequlity.* 2nd ed. Oxford: Clarendon Press.

Sen, Amartya K. 1999. *Development as Freedom.* New York; Knopf Press.

Shah, Shekhar, 1999. "Coping with Natural Disasters: The 1998 Floods in Bangladesh." Seminar paper presented in June to the World Bank, Washington, D.C.

Shapiro, Gilbert, and John Markoff. 1997. "A Matter of Definition." In Carl W. Roberts, ed., *Text Analysis for the Social Sciences.* Mahwah, N.J. Lawrence Erlbaum Assoicates.

Silverman, David. 1993. *Interpreting Qualitative Data; Methods for Analyzing Talk, Text and Interaction.* Thousand Oaks, Calif.: Sage Publications.

Srinivas, Smitra. 1999. *Social Protection for Women Workers in the Informal Economy.* Draft. Washington, D.C.: World Bank and Geneva; International Labour Office.

Standing, Guy. 1999. "Global Feminization through Flexible Labor: A Theme Revisited." *World Development* 3(27): 583-602.

Stone, P.J., D. C. Dunphy, M.S. Smith, and D.M. Ogilvie. 1966. *The General Inquirer; A Computer Approach to Content Analysis.* Cambridge: MIT Press.

Strauss, Anselm. 1987. *Qualitative Analysis for Social Scientists.* New York: Cambridge University Press.

Tarrow, Sidney. 1994. *Power in Movement; Social Movements, Collective Action and Politics.* Cambridge, U.K.: Cambridge University Press.

Tendler, Judith. 1997. *Good Government in the Tropics. Baltimore,* Md.: Johns Hopkins University Press.

Towsen, Peter. 1971. *The Concept of Poverty.* London: Heinemann Educational.

Tripp, Aili Mari. 1992. "The Impact of Crisis and Economic Reform on Women in Urban Tanzania." In Lourdes Beneria and Shelly Feldman, (eds.) *Unequal Burden: Economic Crises, Persistent Poverty, and Women's Work.* Boulder, Colo.: Westiview Press.

Uphoff, Norman, Milton J. Esman, and Anirudh Krishna. 1997. *Reasons for Success; Learning from Instructive Experiences in Rural Development.* West Hartford, Conn.: Kumarian Press.

Uphoff, Norman. 1986. *Local Institutional Development; An Analytical Sourcebook with Cases.* West Harford, Conn.: Kumarian Press.

Visaria, Leela. 1999. "Violence against Women in India: Evidence from Rural Gurjarat." In *Domestic Violence in India: A Summary Report of Three Studies.* Washington, D.C.; International Center for Research on Women.

Weber, Robert Philip. 1990. *Basic Content Analysis.* 2nd ed. Newbury Park, Calif.: Sage Publications.

WHO (World Health Organization). 1997. *Violence against Women.* Geneva.

Woolcock, Michael, and Deepa Narayan. 2000. "Social Capital: Implications for Development Theory, Research, and Policy." *World Bank Research Observer* 15(2), Washington, D.C.: World Bank.

Woolcock, Michael. 1998. "Social Capital and Economic Development: Toward a Theoretical Synthesis and Policy Framework." *Theory and Society 27*(2): 151-208.

World Bank. 1996a. *From Plan to Market: World Development Report 1996.* Washington, D.C.

World Bank. 1996b. *Sourcebook on Participation.* Washington, D.C.

World Bank. 1997a. *Poverty Assessment: A Process Review.* Operations Evaluation Department Document 15881. Washington, D.C.

World Bank. 1997b. *World Development Report 1997: The State in a Changing World.* New York: Oxford University Press (for the World Bank).

World Bank. 1998. *World Development Indicators.* Washington, D.C.

World Bank. 1999. *World Development Indicators.* Washington, D.C.

World Bank. 2000. *Poverty Trends and Voices of the Poor.* Poverty Reduction Group. Washington, D.C.

Wratten, Ellen, 1995. "Conceptualizing Urban Poverty." *Environment and Urbanization* 7: 11-36.

# Index

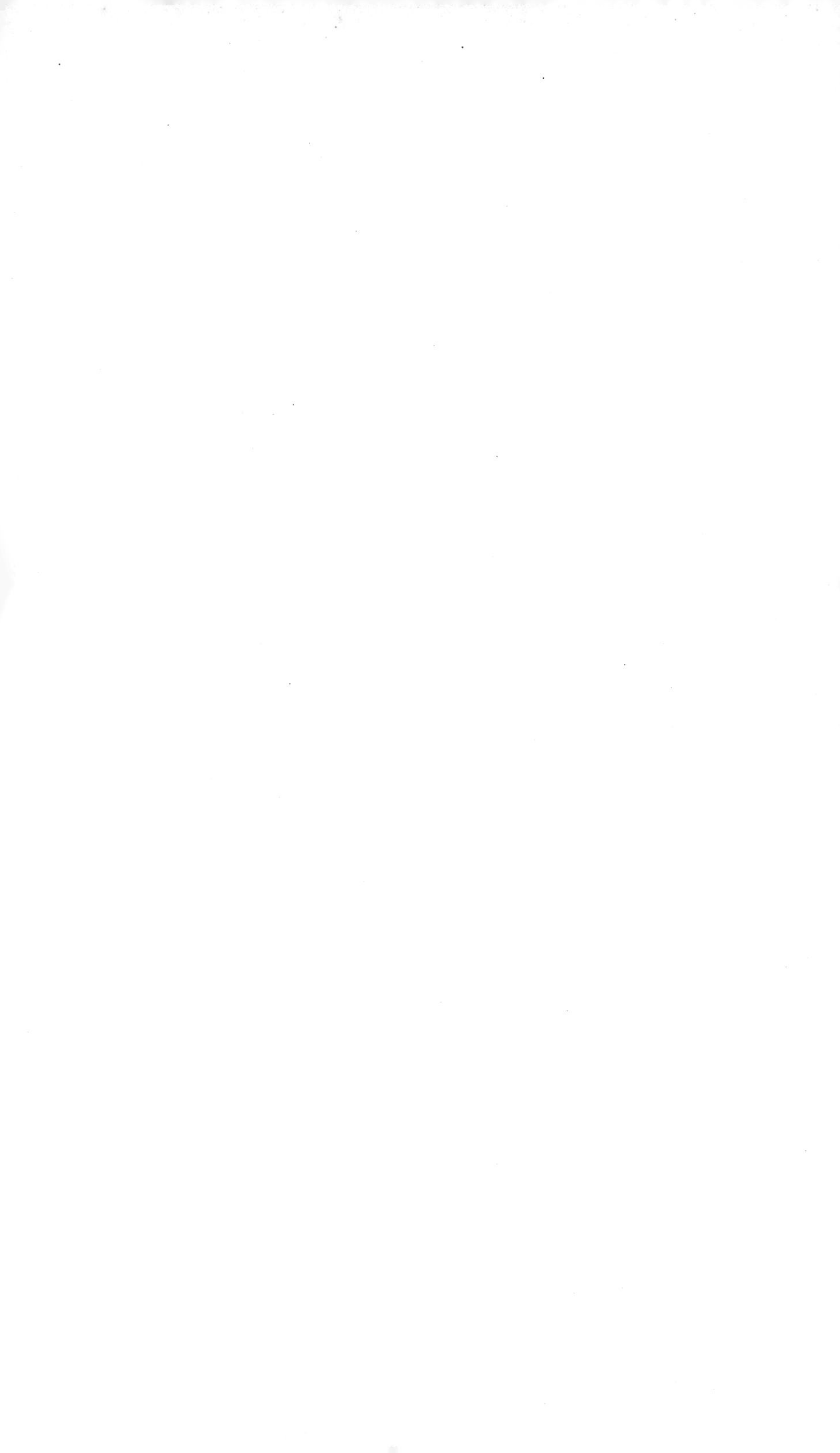